T0296153

MEDICAL PRACTITIONERS
1529–1725

Medical Practitioners in the Diocese of London, Licensed under the Act of 3 Henry VIII, C. 11

An Annotated List 1529–1725

by

J. HARVEY BLOOM, M.A., Hon. F.S.G.

and

R. RUTSON JAMES, F.R.C.S.

CAMBRIDGE
AT THE UNIVERSITY PRESS
1935

CAMBRIDGE
UNIVERSITY PRESS

University Printing House, Cambridge CB2 8BS, United Kingdom

Published in the United States of America by Cambridge University Press, New York

Cambridge University Press is part of the University of Cambridge.

It furthers the University's mission by disseminating knowledge in the pursuit of
education, learning and research at the highest international levels of excellence.

www.cambridge.org
Information on this title: www.cambridge.org/9781107425941

© Cambridge University Press 1935

This publication is in copyright. Subject to statutory exception
and to the provisions of relevant collective licensing agreements,
no reproduction of any part may take place without the written
permission of Cambridge University Press.

First published 1935
First paperback edition 2014

A catalogue record for this publication is available from the British Library

ISBN 978-1-107-42594-1 Paperback

PREFACE

The following list of those licensed to practise in the Diocese of London under the Act of 3 Hen. VIII, c. 11 is drawn from various sources and is arranged in two sections.

The first section contains in chronological order the names entered in the Books of the Vicars-General of the See of London, now housed in the Principal Probate Registry, Somerset House, and, in like manner, the entries in the later books still at St Paul's. The second section is derived from the bundles of original papers also preserved at St Paul's, and here the names are arranged in alphabetical order. An Appendix contains a selection of the more important documents, which have been transcribed as examples of the *modus operandi*, and a list of the Vicars-General of the See who acted as the bishop's commissioners.

We are under an obligation to the Registrar of the Bishop of London, Mr Charles Lee, and to Mr Cave, the chief clerk, and his assistants for their kindly aid and courtesy; and we are specially grateful to Mr Frank Marcham, who has placed his unrivalled knowledge of medieval London and the records in general at our disposal without stint. Without his help the book would have been far less complete than it is.

It must not be assumed that this book contains the names of all practitioners in the diocese. The Royal College of Physicians was clearly outside the provisions of the Act; and, with regard to the surgeons and barber-surgeons, the practice of obtaining a licence from the episcopal authority was certainly not universal.

Young, in the *Annals of the Barber-Surgeons*, thinks that it applied only to some surgeons who were not free of the Company, but the text does not support this view.

He says, 'In some cases the Bishop licensed surgeons, without reference to the Company, and thousands have been licensed by the Company, without regard to the Bishop,...the practice certainly varying with the times'.

The annotations are drawn from the usual accepted sources, Young's *Annals* having proved a mine of information. We wish to state that we have not thought it necessary to refer at length to such well-known men as Clowes, Bernard, Cheselden and Dickins, about whom much is already known. To Mr C. J. S. Thompson's *The Quacks of Old London* we are indebted for facts about T. Saffold and Major Choke.

We are also indebted to Dr G. A. Auden and, through him, to the late Dr Evelyn of York, for information about Alexius Vodka. To the Cambridge University Press we are indebted for kindly consideration and assistance.

J. H. B.
R. R. J.

London
December 1934

INTRODUCTION

The object of the present treatise is to collect, in a more or less orderly manner, the little we have been enabled to find concerning the manner in which the bishops of London handled their great and serious responsibility respecting the licensing of medical practitioners under the Act of Parliament cited as 3 Hen. VIII, c. 11. This act has been frequently printed, not only in the various editions of the *Statutes at Large* but in such works of reference as Willcock's *Laws relating to the Medical Profession*, and Sir D'Arcy Power's more modern work. It is, however, needful to repeat it in this place, that its exact terms may more readily be referred to. It reads:

Forasmoche as the science and connyng of Physyke (and Surgerie) to the perfecte knowlege whereof bee requisite bothe grete lernynge and ripe experience, ys daily within this Royalme exercised by a grete multitude of ignoraunt persones, of whom the grete partie have no manner of insight in the same nor in any other kynde of lernyng, some also (can) no letters on the boke so far furth, that common artificers as Smythes, Wevers, and Women, boldely and customably take upon them grete cures and thyngys of grete difficultie, in tha whiche they partely use Socery and which crafte, partly applie such medicyne unto the disease as be verey noyous and nothing metely, therefore, to the high displeasure of God, great infamy of the faculty, and the grevous hurte damage and distruccion of many of the Kyng's liege people, most especially of them that cannot descerne the uncunnyng from the cunnyng. Be it therefore to the surety and comfort of all manner of people by the auctoritie of thys present parliament enacted, That noo person within the citie of London nor within VII myles of the same, take upon hym to exercise and occupie as a Phisicion or Surgion, except he be first examined, and approved, and admitted, by the bishop of London, or by the Dean of Poules for the time beyng, callyng to hym or them iiii Doctours of Phisyk, and for Surgerie other expert persons in that facultie, And for the first examynacion such as they shall thynk convenient, and afterward alway iiii of them that have been so approved, upon the payn of forfeytour for every moneth that they doo occupie as Phisicions or Surgeons, not admitted nor examined, after the tenour of thys Acte, of V li. to be employed the oon half thereof to thuse of our Soveraign Lord the Kyng, and the other half to any person that wyll sue for it by accion of dette, in which no wageour of Lawe nor perteccion shalbe allowed. And all over thys that noo person out of the seide Citie and precincte of vii myles of the same, except he have been as is seid before approved in the same, take upon him to exercise and occupie as a Phisicion or Surgeon in any diocesse within thys Royalme, but if he be first examined and approved by the Bishop of the same diocesse or beyng out of the diocesse, by his Vicar Generall, either of them callyng to them such expert persons in the seid faculties as there discrecion shall thynk convenyent, and gyffyng ther letters testimonials under their Sealle, to hym that they shall soe approue, upon the like payn to them that occupie the contarie to thys acte as is above seid to be levyed and employed after the fourme before expressed, provided alway that thys acte nor any thyng therin conteyned be prejudiciall to the Universities of Oxford and Cantebrigge or either of them, or to any privilegys graunted to them.

(*Statutes of the Realm*, ed. 1817, vol. 3, p. 32.)

It is no part of our purpose to enter minutely into a discussion of any previous efforts to regulate the practice of either medicine or surgery; but it is needful to remind the readers of our treatise that there were not only schools of medicine at the two universities, but that as far back as 1368 the city of London had made a tentative attempt to license

(*Craft of Surgery*, F. South, ed. D'A. Power), and from an early date a Mystery of Barbours existed in the city, and obtained a charter from Edward IV (Willcock, p. clxvii) in which those members of the Mystery using the faculty of chirurgery are supported against the foreign surgeons, who were not freemen of the city. There was also a less lawful company of pure surgeons, and these became so powerful that a union of the two became a necessity. This union was carried into effect by a statute put forth in 1540–41 cited as 32 Hen. VIII, c. 42. This union continued until the Act of Parliament, cited as 18 Geo. II, c. 15 (1744–5), separated them into two distinct companies once more, by which time the Bishop of London had ceased to exercise his authority under the Act of Henry VIII.

Under a charter bearing date 15 August 5 Charles (1629),

It was granted that no person or persons whatsoever for the future,...shall use or exercise the said art or science of surgery within our said cities of London and Westminster or either of them, or within the distance of seven miles of the said city of London, for his or their private lucre...unless the said person ...be first examined in the presence of two or more of the masters or governors of the mystery or commonalty aforesaid, who for the time shall be, by four or more examiners of the same society for the time being, so as aforesaid elected and appointed, and by public letters testimonial of the same masters or governors, under their common seal, approved of and admitted to exercise the art or science of Surgery, according to the laws and statutes of this our kingdom...

which is as much of the wording of the charter as concerns the present purpose.

Our object has been to examine what evidences remain between the years 1512 and 1740 to illustrate the working of the Act of Henry VIII within the Diocese of London.

Unfortunately it is not until the year 1529 that any document remains. In that year we have a record of the negotiation for letters testimonial for a John Johnson of St Clement Danes. Since this is the earliest document so far discovered it is worth study. In this case the applicant was presented to the bishop, in his palace by St Paul's, by two doctors of medicine, and the masters of the Mystery of Surgeons, apparently after examination by the four other surgeons whose names are given, who declare him 'expert and able to exercise the art of chirurgery' (see App., I).

Yet more precise in wording are the letters testimonial granted to Thomas Skoes on 9 August 1555. He was brought before the Lord Bishop in the upper gallery of his episcopal palace by three qualified medical men, Thomas Vycary, George Holland, and George Geen, who certified that they had diligently examined him and certain others named, whereupon the bishop decreed that letters testimonial should be made and sealed according to the statute (see App., II). This was done before Bishop Edmund (Bonner) in person, and Robert Johnson, notary public, his registrar.

In another example dated 8 February 1562, Patrick Sele and John Willoughbye, a clerk, came to the house of the Vicar-General (Master Huycke) and brought with them written proof that the four ex-

4

aminers appointed were satisfied, and accordingly letters testimonial were issued under the episcopal seal (see App., III).

In this year an example survives of even more formal proceedings. William Clowes (the celebrated surgeon) is the candidate. He came before the bishop's chancellor (Master Edward Stanhope) in his chambers, and there in the presence of William Blackwell, notary, produced letters, signed and sealed, from the masters of his mystery, testifying that their examiners had satisfied themselves that the candidate was qualified by practice and experience to receive letters testimonial from the bishop, which letters were duly granted after Clowes had taken his oath of allegiance to the Queen's majesty (see App., IV).

A variant in the procedure is found in 1586 when Roger Gyankins, in his own person, appeared before the chancellor and his notary, and brought with him letters testimonial from four masters of his company certifying his ability as a surgeon. Whereupon, his efficiency being established, the Vicar-General ordered letters testimonial to be prepared and sealed according to the statute, and a copy of them drawn up to be kept in the registry, and the originals to be handed back to Roger.

This leads to the entry in the Vicar-General's books in stately English, and thus for the first time we see entered the full text of these grants.

Such a letter is addressed to all Christian people. It is an open letter sent out unsealed, to be read by all. The bishop sends his greeting in our Lord God everlasting, and then commences a preamble, citing the reasons why such powers had been granted to him and why they were needed, namely, 'because of the presumptious unpunished boldness of uncunninge chirurgeons' and for 'avoyding grevous hurtes and jeopardies whiche daylie happen' from that cause. The bishop claims that such power was conferred upon him by statute, within the city of London and seven miles round, that he has called in four qualified men, chirurgeons admitted by the bishops his predecessors, who have examined the applicant (Hugh Lingen) and found him 'righte hable and sufficiente to occupie and exercise the said facultie and science of chirurgerie', and have accordingly admitted him, he having first sworn 'on the holie evangelistes' before the chancellor and registrar, to obey 'the Queenes moste excellente Majestie'. The seal of the chancellor is the seal *ad causas* used for less important documents. The formal date is added, viz. 26 February 1588, in the twelfth year of the bishop's consecration.

It is not difficult to perceive that the claims of the Bishop of London, as stated in this last formal document, ran counter to the claims of the Mystery of Barbers and Chirurgeons of London, who, for a long time previously, had allowed certain freemen of their company to practise chirurgery within the city and its precinct.

There is plenty of evidence of extreme ill-feeling between the two authorities, of which more will be said later.

On 16 August 1577 Edmund, Bishop of Norwich, granted letters testimonial to one John Croppe of Norwich, who afterwards moved to London and produced this document to support his claim for a similar one from his new diocesan. This was granted to him on 1 February 1590, both documents being entered in the Vicar-General's book in full.

It is not until the reign of James I that there is any hint that orthodoxy was a necessary and important part if the candidate wished for permission to 'occupie his arte'. But in 1618, in the case of Robert Luskin of Harwich, we find such a clause inserted. We should have judged that the conformity of Master Vodka was a matter solely for the Archbishop of York, and the reason for Laud's interference does not appear, but it seems he took some steps to ensure that Vodka's profession did not begin and end with attending prayers in Laud's chapel. We fear that at this date the theology of an applicant far outweighed in importance his skill in his science, and Vodka's was not an isolated case. It continued long after the Restoration, and varied to suit the views of the time.

The ecclesiastical authorities ceased to function from July 1640 to April 1660. In the interval much had happened prejudicial to acts of a chancellor and indeed to the bishop himself, but it in no way concerns us. When, however, the curtain lifts, we find files of documents in the archive rooms of St Paul's. These original papers vary greatly in character, and hardly ever cover quite the same ground. Some are attractively human in their interest, and others purely formal; in this class may be placed the stately Latin certificates emanating from the universities, the College of Physicians, the Company of Barber-Surgeons, and, most unexpectedly, from Sion College. In the former class we must reckon the personal letters from the clergy and churchwardens, which form a sort of covering letter, supporting the certificate of those local medical men who bear witness to the applicant's skill. Such letters are generally from outlying places, and one at least pleads the impossibility of fulfilling the requirement of medical attestation, because none existed between Colchester and Ipswich.

The procedure at this date seems to be that an applicant's papers were read by the chancellor or his surrogate, and assent in the form *fiat lic*. written at the foot, after which the clerks drew up the licence and filed away the papers. There is no longer any evidence that the candidates came before the bishop, or that their medical supporters did so either. The chancellor, in fact, acted as commissioner for the bishop.

Members of the universities holding medical degrees had always been exempt from the bishop's jurisdiction, but even so there exist rare cases, as may be seen from the lists, and the same applies to fellows of the College of Physicians. The bulk of the licences are granted to freemen, or at least members of the barber-surgeons, and this in spite of the friction already hinted at between the company and the bishop. In the end the accidental preservation of a letter shows that some official with a singular lack

8

of tact tried to force all surgeons holding the company's diploma to attend the Visitation of the Bishop, a claim that was keenly resented, and it is small wonder that within a few years the registrar had to be content to take the sum of £5 yearly, in lieu of issuing any surgical licences at all. There does not seem to have been any repeal of the Act of Henry VIII. It died apparently from inanition—a useless anachronism.

In studying these later papers, it must be evident that it was only those who had been through a long course of apprenticeship to a recognised medical man, seven years seems usual, and had in their own case proved by their practice that they were sufficiently skilled, who could stand much chance of a licence. Many others of whom we know nothing may have applied, but there is no evidence for or against it. The bishop, anxious to fill a need in a remote country place, was not perchance too exacting, and once sure of his orthodoxy, coupled with some little training, the applicant might well be passed.

To sum up, Henry VIII must have the honour of enjoining a system regulating doctors of medicine and masters in surgery, which covered the whole country. He chose as its medium the organisation of the Church, since it reached everywhere and was splendidly efficient; moreover, the connection between physical and spiritual sickness is not difficult to discover. In the hour of birth with its Sacrament of Baptism, and in the hour of death and all the time between, the help of medical and clerical advice was

9

very near. The Church had the last word in marriage, testaments, and so forth, it was only fitting, so Henry would argue, that medical men should be under its control.

All would have been well but for the greed of the faculty. Henry had followed up the Act in question by another cited as 5 Hen. VIII, c. 6, freeing surgeons from serving on juries and as constables. And later still, 32 Hen. VIII, c. 42, the King united the ancient Company of Barbers, established by letters patent of Edward IV, 24 February 1461–2, with the incorporate surgeons, and both were exempted from bearing of armour, inquests, and watches, etc. The so-called 'Quacks' Charter', cited as 34–35 Hen. VIII, c. 8, enacts that

the company and fellowship of surgeons of London, minding only their own lucres, and nothing the profit, or ease of the diseased or patient, have soe troubled and vexed divers honest persons, as well men as women, whom God hath endued with the knowledge of the nature of...certain herbs...and yet the said persons have not taken any thing for their pains or cunning but have ministerd the same to poor people only for neighbourhood and God's sake...and it is now well known that the surgeons admitted, will do no cure to any person, but where they know they shall be rewarded. This act allows such persons to prescribe and treat such things as sore breasts, a web* in the eye, uncomes† of hands, burnings, scaldings, sore mouths, the stone, strangury, saucelim,‡ morphew,§ and such like diseases.

An important charter was granted by the King on 15 August 1639. It placed all the surgeons in London

* Corneal nebula.   † Whitlow.
‡ Chaucer's saucefleme, a scurvy face.   § Scurf on the skin.

and seven miles round under the control of the Mystery of Barbers and Surgeons of London, and forbade any to practise within those limits without examination by the company's elected examiners, under a certificate sealed with their common seal, under a penalty of £5 for each such offence.

Previous to this charter, it seems that the bishops sometimes appointed for their examiners only those who had been admitted by their predecessors.

No specially eminent names are to be found in these papers except as making the required certificate of competency. Among such may be mentioned Sir Hans Sloane, John Evelyn the Diarist, and the infamous Titus Oates, who barefacedly styles himself B.A. of Cambridge, which he was not.

A last word must be said on a subject about which there is nothing in the Act of Parliament. We mean the licensing of midwives, a part of the bishop's work to which especial attention is paid. This is no doubt due to their importance in view of the prompt administration of baptism, if danger to the infant's life seemed to be imminent. In order to make our treatise as complete as possible a few examples are given in the Appendix to illustrate the form of licence. In the case of these women, four or more other women, experienced in midwifery, gave evidence before the bishop or the chancellor that the candidate had not only experience, but had been skilful in bringing a child into the world. It follows that she had to be of good repute and orthodox in her faith.

SECTION I

Letters testimonial and other documents contained in the books of the Vicars-General of the Bishops of London now preserved in the principal probate registry, Somerset House.

1529. JOHNSON, JOHN, of St Clement without the barrs of the New Temple. Presented to the bishop in his palace of London, by Master Edward Fynche and Arthur Malachias, Doctors in Medicine. Robert Beverley, Thomas Gybson, John Mownford, and Thomas Powting, Wardens of the Mystery of Chirurgeons. Examiners: Edward Classehead, Baldewyn Kyrkeby, John Taller, and Christopher Dixson, chirurgeons, 10 Dec.

Foxford, f. 203d.

Perhaps of St Margaret, New Fish Street; Will proved 20 June 1533. *Com. Lond. Tunstall, 214.*

GARLAND, RALPH.

Warden, Barber-Surgeons' Company, 1530, 1533, 1536.

SUTTON, THOMAS.

Warden, Barber-Surgeons' Company, 1528.

YOUNG, JOHN.

Possibly Senior Warden, Barber-Surgeons' Company, 1527.

WHYTE, CHARLES.

SPENSER, WILLIAM.

Possibly William Spencer, Warden, Barber-Surgeons' Company, 1537.

JONSON, MATHEW.

Matthew Johnson, Warden, Barber-Surgeons' Company,
1550. In a list of 19 Sept. 1552 Johnson is dismissed of
his livery because 'he ys not habull' (solvent).

ANGIR, JOHN.

Possibly John Anger, Liveryman of the Company in 1537.

MONE, THOMAS.

Liveryman of the Company, 1537.

WYLSON, THOMAS.

Thomas Wilson, Liveryman of the Company, 1537.

BOWLING, CHRISTOPHER.

Probably the Christopher Bolling, Liveryman of the
Company in 1537.

SPYGHALL, ROBERT.

Probably Robert Sprignell, Warden of the Barber-
Surgeons' Company, 1540, 1547, 1551, and Master, 1554.
Donor of a cup to the Company.

NEWTON, HENRY.

HORSLEY, JOHN, of Chelchister (Colchester).

All of whom were granted letters testimonial 24 Jan.
1529–30 after examination by Thomas Vicary, Thomas
Gybson, Henry Baldewyne, and John Alyef, and allowed
to practise chirurgery.   *Foxford, f. 207d.*

STERR (STARR in margin), JOHN, chirurgeon. Exam.
as above, dated 21 April 1531.   *Ibid. f. 209.*

ROGERS, THOMAS, of the precinct of St Martin le Grand
(*magni*), surgeon. Exam. as above, 13 June 1531.
Ibid. f. 232.

HATTON, CHRISTOPHER, surgeon (?), no parish. Exam.
as last, 17 June 1531.   *Ibid.*

13

CUTHBERTH, THOMAS, chirurgeon. Exam. Thomas Vicary, John Ayleffe, George Holand, and John Enderby, chirurgeons, 22 Jan. 1534–5.

Legacy of silver instruments and a salvatory by Will of Henry Baldewyn, 1534. *Com. Lond. Tunstall, 228.*

WODE, JAMES, as last.

CRAGELL, JOHN, as last.

Will (*Com. Lond. Story, 162*) proved 11 Sept. 1545. Of St John's Walbroke. Legacies to godson, 'towards his scole'; overseer, James Thompson, 'sometime my Master'. Residue to wife.

BOWYNE, JOHN, as last.

Note. These four names form a short list all examined by the same four surgeons and admitted on 22 Jan. Two of them, Thomas Cutbert and John Cragell, were freemen of their Company in 1537, while James Wood was Warden in 1551, 1557 and 1560, and Master in 1566. *Foxford, f. 243.*

SELE, PATRICK. In the presence of the chancellor and registrar, Master Huycke and Peter Johnson, after exam. by George Hollande, Richard Ferrys, George Gynne, and Thomas Gale, 8 Feb. 1562.

WILLOUGHBY, JOHN, clerk. On the same day after exam. by the said surgeons. *Huicke, f. 72.*

SKOES, THOMAS. Admitted in the upper gallery of the bishop's palace, 9 Aug. 1555.

UPTON, RYCHARD.

Junior Warden of the Barbers and Surgeons of London, 1574; complained of by Edward Browne, a bricklayer, in 1572 for taking money to cure the *morbus gallicus* and failing to do so.

WEST, JOHN.

Junior Warden of the said Company, 1563. Fined in 1551 for 'speking opprobryous wordes against John Androwson in the presence of the masters'.

MASON, JOHN.

Junior Warden of the Company, 1575. Apprenticed to Nicholas Alcocke, who left him some of his books.

WEST, ROBERT.

WATER, THOMAS.

WARNER, THOMAS.

PYKE, ROBERT, surgeon of St Katheryns.

BACTERE, JOHN, clerk.

All of whom after exam. by the last-named examiners, 16 July 1555. The form of admission of Thomas Skoes is entered in Latin. The examiners appeared in person and letters testimonial were accordingly decreed. 9 Aug.

All, save John Bactere, were citizens and barber-surgeons of London.

CROWE, WILLIAM.

Warden of the Company 1576, 1579, 1582; Master in 1585.

FIELDE, JOHN.

Barber-surgeon of London. Warden of his Company in 1568-9, 1574; Master in 1577. Apprenticed to Richard Ferris, serjeant-surgeon.

PYCKTON, HENRY.

An apprentice to Thomas Vicary, and a legatee under his will.

TRAPPY, HENRY.

BLUNDYE, ALARD, a stranger, surgeon of London.

WILKYNSON, WILLIAM, of Dunstable, barber-surgeon.

MYNAS, PETER, of London, barber-surgeon.

The above seven persons were granted letters testimonial, after examination by Thomas Vycary, Richard Ferrys, George Holland, and George Gynne, 29 July 1558. The original notification is sewn into the register.

Croke, f. 305.

Sele, Patrick. *Vide supra.*

John Willoughby, clerk. *Vide supra.*

These two persons were admitted to practise, in the house of the Vicar-General, Master Huycke, in the presence of Peter Johnson the registrar, 8 Feb. 1562–3, after exhibiting a schedule signed by George Hollande, Richard Ferrys, George Gynne, and Thomas Gale, examiners.

Huicke, f. 72.

Hollingworth, Robert, of Colchester, chirurgeon. Admitted 23 Aug. 1564, on exhibiting a schedule signed by George Holland, Thomas Gale, and Robert Balthropp. *Ibid. f. 93.*

Slade, William, chirurgeon. Received letters testimonial, 25 Jan. 1570–1, after exhibiting a schedule signed by Robert Balthroppe, Alexander Mason, Thomas Bayley, and Robert Modsley, examiners.

Clowes, William, citizen and chirurgeon. Was admitted at the request of the Queen, 26 March 1580, in the chambers of Edward Stanhope, official principal, in the presence of William Blackwell, notary, after examination by Robert Muddesley, John Field, William Bovie, and John Yates, examiners, attested by William Clovey, barber of London, William Eden, clerk of the Company, William Bovee, William Crowe and Thomas Birde, Masters of the same.

William Clowes was a famous Elizabethan surgeon. He was born about 1540, the son of Thomas Clowes of Kingsbury, in the county of Warwick, and later of London. He studied his art under George Keble, and saw service in both the army and navy. He settled in London and was living in St Olave's, Old Jewry, in 1595, where his daughter had a licence to marry William Gregory of St Martin's, Outwich, 5 July in that year. He was surgeon of St Bartholomew's Hospital and died in 1604.

16

GALE, WILLIAM, chirurgeon, citizen and barber-surgeon of London. Received a licence to practise his art, 7 Nov. 1583, after examination by Thomas Bankes, Leonard Coxe, Richard Wood, William Crowe, John Yates, and William Bovey.   *Stanhope, i, f. 2.*

He was Warden of his Company in 1583, 1590, and Master in 1595, and died holding that office for the second time, 19 Nov. 1610. By his first wife he had five sons and eight daughters. He was buried at Monken Hadley, co. Middlesex, where there is a brass to his memory. He was aged about 70 at his death.

WOODE, RICHARD, citizen and chirurgeon of London. Licensed on the same day.   *Ibid.*

Warden of his Company 1585, 1588, Master, 1599.

BURGIS, JOHN, chirurgeon of London. Licensed 27 Aug. 1584, on the testimony of the examiners of the Mystery of Barbers and Surgeons, whose names are not given, but a copy of which was at the time preserved in the Registry.   *Ibid. f. 24.*

Probably that John Burgess who was Warden of the Company in 1593 and 1598.

GRAYE, SAMUEL, of St Sepulchre, London, chirurgeon. Licensed after examination by Robert Mudesley, William Bovey, Henry Rankyn, and John Heysey, examiners of the said Company, 17 March 1584–5.

GYANKINS, ROGER, citizen and chirurgeon of London. Granted letters testimonial under the hand and seal of Edward Stanhope, in the presence of William Sadler, notary publique, on certificates of Robert Muddesley, William Bovye, John Yates, and John Hasye, then Masters of the Mystery of Chirurgeons. A copy being made for the use of the office, the originals were returned.   *Ibid. f. 138.*

Possibly Roger Jenkins, Warden of his Company 1608. 1611, 1614. Free of the Weavers' Company, and admitted

'Bro^r in the practize of surgery'. He paid £10 for his livery. '9, July 1607, this day R. G. was presented before the Deane of Pawles.'

LINGEN, HUGH, of St Buttolphe's without Aldgate, chirurgeon. The full form of admission in English, dated 26 Feb. 1588, after examination by Master Leonard Coxe, Richard Wood, William Borne, and George Denham, chirurgeons appointed by 'our predecessors bishops of London', admitted after being sworn on the 'holie evangelistes to the supremacie of the Queene's moste excellente Majestie'.

Stanhope, i, f. 257.

WESTE, THOMAS, of St Andrew in Holborne, chirurgeon. Licence being granted to practise and exercise the art of chirurgery within the diocese of London, 16 Dec. 1589. Testimonial of the examiners in this case, John Heysey, William Boovey, Richard Wistowe, and William Gale, 'examiners of that art within the city of London and seven miles round'.

Ibid. f. 316 (Latin).

WOODE, THOMAS, of Chelmesford, chirurgeon. Admitted 12 April 1591, 'having received sufficient testimony from Thomas Annatt, Robert Turner, and George Chapman, practitioners in surgery'.

Stanhope, ii, f. 27 (English).

HOBBES, THOMAS, chirurgeon. 'Negotium' 11 Dec. 1594 before Master Edward Stanhope and Thomas Pell, notary public, when he appeared in person and exhibited letters under the hands of William Clowes, John Nusam, and John Izard, then Masters of the Mystery, and examiners of the surgeons of London, etc. *Ibid. f. 201 (Latin).*

CROPPE, JOHN, of Norwich, chirurgeon. Who produced letters testimonial of Edmund (Scambler), Bishop of Norwich, granting him a licence to practise in and through our diocese, 16 Aug. 1577 (Latin). On the strength of which, Croppe having come to London, the bishop having approved, admits him, after taking the usual oath, 1 Feb. 1590. This is in English and signed Will. Blakwell, deputatus.

Stanhope, ii, f. 20.

John Crop, physician, owned the advowson of the church of St Peter Hungate, Norwich, 1615–27 (*Blomfield and Parkin, Hist. of Norfolk, vol. iv, p. 331*).

PORTER, PETER, of Le Savoy, co. Middlesex, chirurgeon. Admitted 8 Oct. 1596, after producing letters testimonial subscribed by William Bovie, Henry Ranckin, Richard Wood, and William Gale, examiners of chirurgeons of London. *Stanhope, iii, f. 115.*

Perhaps that Peter Porter who was a Warden of the Barber-Surgeons' Company from 1617 to 1619.

PARRIE, ALEXANDER, of London, chirurgeon. Admitted by Edward Stanhope, LL.D., in the voidance of the See, 'having received sufficient testimony from William Goodowrus, serjeant-chirurgeon to his Majesty, William Bovie, Richard Wood, and William Gale, examiners', 1 April 1597. *Ibid. f. 141.*

LAMBERT, PETER, clerk, M.A., curate of the parish church of Braxted Magna, co. Essex. Licensed 'ad dandum et ministrandum medicinas et medicamenta et salubria ac consilium' to all and singular within our diocese, dated 3 Dec. 1597.

Stanhope, v. f. 10 (Latin).

JOHNSON, JOHN, of London, chirurgeon. Admitted on sufficient testimony of Richard Wood, William Gale, John Izard, and Lewes Atmer, examiners appointed in chirurgery, 12 Dec. 1598. On which day John Johnson of St Dunstan's in the West appeared and exhibited a certificate, under the common seal of the Surgeons' Hall subscribed by John Leycock, John

Burges, Thomas Thorney, and Robert Johnson, masters, attesting the abovesaid examination.
Stanhope, iv, f. 92.

LOVEDAY, SALAMON, of Braintry, in the county of Essex, chirurgeon, 'havinge received sufficiente testimonie bothe of the good liefe and honest conversation...and likewise of his approved skill and knowledge in the Science and Arte of Chirurgery, doe approve and admitte him...and have caused the seale of our Chancelour to be sett to these presentes', dated 3 Sept. 1602. *Stanhope, v, f. 75.*

FOSTER, WILLIAM, 'a free brother of the Mistery of Barbers and Surgeons of the Citty of London, sometyme Master of Anatomy in the Arte of Chirurgery, Approved to be an hable and sufficiente surgeon, on testimony of Thomas Thorney, William Martin, Edward Rodes, and Thomas Martin Masters of the said Mistery, after examination by Thomas Thorney, William Martyn, Richard Wood, and Christopher Fredrick, Masters in that Arte'. Signed by Stanhope and Will. Blackwell. *Ibid. f. 225.*

Perhaps that William Foster who was fined in Sept. 1606 for 'his evil practize upon his patient, being a servaunt of my Lord grace of Cant.' He was defrauded of another patient by one of his fellows in December in the same year.

NICHOLSON, WILLIAM, M.A. Admitted to practise medicine after exhibiting letters testimonial from Robert Ram, S.T.P., and taking the oath of supremacy, dated 6 Nov. 1609. He 'allegavit in super se nunc intendere vitam agere in practica ejusdem'.
Crompton, f. 100 (Latin).

HIGGINSON, LAURENCE, of St Martin's within Ludgate, London. *Edwards, f. 8.*

Citizen and barber-chirurgeon, whose wife, Anne, was licensed to practise midwifery, 1611.

20

PARNELL, WILLIAM, of Endfield, Middlesex. A brief note that he was licensed to practise medicine, 22 Feb. –3. 1622   *Edwards, f. 92.*

LOVEDAY, SALAMON, of Brayntry, chirurgeon. Note of a confirmation of a previous licence (see above) under the hands of Thomas Edwardes and Robert Christian, Deputy Registrar, dated 21 April 1613.
                                                                                      Ibid. f. 96.

TOWE, WILLIAM, of St Albans, surgeon. Note of a licence granted 12 May 1613.   *Ibid. f. 100.*

MATHIE, JOHN, of St Albans (?). Similar note, dated 10 June 1613.   *Ibid. f. 105.*

BARNARDE, ROBERT, of Dunmowe, co. Essex (?). Similar note, dated 24 June 1613.   *Ibid. f. 106.*

LUSKINS, JOHN, of (Bishop's) Stortford, co. Herts, M.A. Admitted to practise medicine and chirurgery, 6 Dec. 1615. A brief note.   *Ibid. f. 196.*

LUSKIN, ROBERT, of Harwich. Licence (full text in Latin) by John King, Bishop of London, to practise medicine and chirurgery, 'the whilst he carries himself honestly and prudently'. Under the seal of the Vicar-General in that part used, dated (blank) Nov. 1618.   *Marten, i, f. 102.*

TILLIARD, ABRAHAM, of St Albans. Note of a licence by George (Abbot), Bishop of London, to practise medicine and chirurgery, dated 8 March 1625–6.
                                                                                Marten, ii, f. 79.

JACOBBE, JOHN, alias UNDERSALIETE, late of Asheford, London. Note of a licence to practise medicine and chirurgery, dated 10 Oct. 1627.   *Ducke, f. 9.*

ANTHONY, CHARLES, M.A. Note of a licence to practise medicine and chirurgery, dated December 1627 (see Section II).

VAN VIVOS, WILLIAM, M.A., of St Peter's in Malden. Note of a licence granted 17 Sept. 1628.

Ducke, f. 43.

ABBIS, THOMAS, of MALDEN. Note of a licence to practise medicine and chirurgery, dated 17 Sept. 1628. *Ibid. f. 44.*

HERBERT, JOHN (no locality). Note of a licence to practise chirurgery, 28 June 1630. *Ibid. f. 95.*

FISHER, EDWARD, of St Sepulchre's, London, Surgeon. Note of admission of his wife, Grace, to practise midwifery, 29 Nov. 1630. *Ibid. f. 98.*

WAGNER, FREDERICK, M.D., of Leigh, co. Essex. Licence to practise medicine, dated 3 Feb. 1630–1.

Ibid. f. 102.

LONE, MASTER JOHN, rector of the church of Shopland, co. Essex. Licence to practise medicine, dated 11 March 1631. *Ibid. f. 132.*
Perhaps of Trinity Hall, Cambridge, born at Rayleigh, co. Essex. M.A. 1613; deacon (London), 1610; aged 24. Curate of Canewdon, co. Essex; priest 1611. *Venn, Alum. Cant.*

KING, WILLIAM, barber-surgeon, of St Lawrence, Old Jurie. Licence (in full) after certificates of Thomas Caldwell, Esq., Andrew Wheatley, John Woodhall, and Daniel Hinxman, Masters of his Company, after examination by Richard Mapes, Richard Cooper, Alexander Barker, and James Mullins, masters in surgery, 15 Nov. 1632. *Ibid. f. 139.*
'Of Catteaton St.' in 1641. City Companies' Poll Tax, 1641. Perhaps the Wm Kinge, surgeon, St Bartholomew's Hospital, 1643–55 (*vide Sir Norman Moore's Hist. St Bartholomew's Hospital, ii, 623 et seq.*).

EATON, HENRY, of St Benet Fincke, chirurgeon.
A member of the livery of the barber-surgeons in 1638. Possibly son of Henry Eaton, citizen and barber-surgeon of

London, who died 1605. He left three daughters 'and the child my wife now goeth with' (Will, *P.C.C. Hayes, 64*). Will (*P.C.C. Harvey, 159*) proved 3 Oct. 1639. Citizen and barber-surgeon of London. Wife, Margaret, executrix. Eldest daughter, Sarah, £100; John, only son, £100, when 21; second daughter, Susan, £100. Brother-in-law and father-in-law, John Woodall, sen. and jun. overseers.

NAPKIN, HUGH, of St Botolph without Aldgate, citizen and chirurgeon.

Also a member of the livery of his company in 1638. Will (*Archd. Lond. Reg. 8, f. 299*) proved 5 Oct. 1639. Rings to various relatives. Wife, Mary, executrix. £3 to those 'members of the livery of my company as shall accompany mee to the grave', for a supper after the funeral.

ARRIS, EDWARD, of St Sepulchre's, London, chirurgeon.

He was son of Jasper Arris, a Warden of the Barber-Surgeons in 1622, and was admitted by patrimony in 1617, after being taught by his father. Held the diploma to practise, 1651. Founded the anatomy lecture named after him, 1645. Died 28 May 1676, aged 85.

The last three were admitted with William King, but the form of licence is in their case omitted.

ROCHESTER, JOHN, of Lawford, Essex, licensed to practise medicine, 16 November 1632. *Ducke, f. 140.*

ALTOFTE, ROBERT, citizen and barber-surgeon of London. Licence (in full) on certificate of John Woodall, Richard Powell, Henry Blackley, and George Priddie, Masters of his Company, after examination by Richard Mapes, Alexander Baker, Richard Watson, and Daniel Hinxman, Masters in Surgery, dated 18 Dec. 1633 and signed by the bishop, William Laud. *Ibid. f. 151d.*

ALLEN, THOMAS, of St Mary le Bowe, barber-surgeon. Licence (in full) upon a certificate from John Molins, Arthur Dowghton, Richard Powell, and John Ward,

Masters of the Company of Barber-Surgeons, after examination by Richard Mapes, Alexander Baker, John Woodall, and Henry Blackley, Masters in Surgery, dated 18 Dec. 1633. *Ibid. f. 152.*

He was a Warden of the said Company in 1649, 1651, 1654, and Master in 1658. A portrait of him hangs in the Election Room in the Company's Hall.

BENNET, WILLIAM, of St Margaret, New Fish Street, London, barber-surgeon. Licence (in full) after certificate from the Masters, etc., named in the last entry. Dated and signed by the bishop as above. *Ibid.*

He was a Warden of the Company in 1647–9, in which latter year he died. Will dated 4 July 1649; proved 1 Jan. 1649/50 (*P.C.C. Pembroke, 2*). To be decently buried. 'Sonn John Bennett, Minister-of-the-Gospel at New Brentford, £10, my gold seale ring with W.B. engraven on it, my stuffe cloake. Daughter, Sarah Cornbee, £10. But if my publiq Faith money and my arreare money that is due, as cann be made appeare by severall papers...in the handes of Anne my wife...if she receive £120, then my son £10 and daughters be made up to £20 each. Daughter Sarah a gold ring. To wife all goodes, lease of house, to be disposed of at her pleasure having by large experience her love and care to my children. To the Company of Barber-Surgeons £5 to make a collation provided that the body of the Livery accompany my body to the grave. Wife, executrix. My loving Master Mr Geo. Dunn and friend, Mr John Cocke, overseers. Wit. John Cocke, Nich. Clagett.'

BULLOCKE, alias BULLUCKE, ROBERT, of St Edmund's, Lombard Street, London, barber-surgeon. After certificate and examination, as in the two last entries, signed and dated as above. *Ducke, f. 152d.*

He was a Warden of the Company in 1652, and Master 1657.

COTTON, LAURENCE, of St Stephen's, Coleman Street, barber-surgeon. Licence (in full) after a certificate from John Woodall, Richard Powell, Henry Blacklie, and George Priddie, Masters of his Company. Examiners: Richard Mapes, Alexander Baker, Richard Wateson, and Daniel Hinxman, Masters in Surgery, dated 18 Dec. 1633. *Ducke, f. 153.*

He was a Warden of the Company 1636–7, and in 1641. Master, 1645. Seems to have disturbed its unity, peace, and amity, by abusing the Master and some of the assistants. He was dismissed from his office as an assistant in 1642, and deposed from the post of examiner.

BOSTOCKE, ENOCH, of St Sepulchre's, London, barber-surgeon. Licence (in full) on certificate of Woodall, etc., as above, and after examination by Mapes, Baker, Arthur Doughton, and Hinxman, dated 26 Feb. 1633–4, signed by the bishop. *Ibid.*

An unsuccessful candidate for the post of surgeon to St Thomas's Hospital in 1633 (*vide Parsons, Hist. St Thomas's Hosp. ii, 43, 58*).

WARD, HUGH, of St Andrew's, Holborn, barber-surgeon. Licence similar to the last, dated 26 Feb. 1633–4.
Ibid. f. 154.

In 1635 Ward was summoned before the Court for absence from lectures but used 'opprobrious language' and defied the Masters, whereupon he was committed to the Compter, but before he reached it drew a knife and 'swoare he would sheathe it in the officer's guttes if he came after him, and soe made his escape'. Two months later he submitted and was fined 40 shillings.

ALLEN, RADULF, Freeman and Professor of Surgery in the City of London. Licence after examination by Mapes, Baker, Richard Watson, and James Molins, dated 20 March 1633–4. *Ibid.*

COCKE, JONATHAN, Chirurgeon of Colchester, licensed to practise medicine and chirurgery throughout the diocese. 5 Sept. 1634. *Ibid. f. 180 d.*

RANFORD, (no christian name), of St Albans, Chirurgeon, licensed, 12 Sept. 1634. *Ibid. f. 183 d.*

WELD, THOMAS, of Tollesbury, co. Essex, chirurgeon. Note of admission, dated 5 Sept. 1634. *Ducke, f. 190.*

LOWE, LAURENCE, barber-surgeon, of St Margaret Pattens, London. Licence after examination by Baker, Molins, Woodall, and Hinxman, dated 20 April 1635. *Ibid. f. 194.*

Possibly Laurence Loe, Warden of his Company in 1653, 1655, 1658, and Master in 1667. He gave a set of marble paving stones to the company for the floor of the hall, which are now in the Monkwell Street entrance. Surgeon, St Thomas's Hospital, 1648. Discharged by Parliament 1649 (*Parsons, Hist. St Thomas's Hosp. ii, 264*).

COLLINS, THOMAS, citizen and barber-surgeon, of St Peter ad vincula, in the Tower of London. Licence, dated 20 April 1635. *Ibid. f. 194.*

He was a Warden of his Company in 1639 and in 1644, Master in 1648.

GRIFFITH, MAURICE, citizen and barber-surgeon of St Martin in the Fields. Note of a licence, dated as in the last. *Ibid.*

A liveryman of the Barber-Surgeons' Company in 1638.

REMMINGTON, ROBERT, of Chelmesford, chirurgeon. Note of admission to practise, 9 Dec. 1634.
Ibid. f. 199.

KING, ROBERT, of the same place. Admitted to practise medicine on the same day. *Ibid.*

KNIGHT, JOHN, of Castle Hedingham, co. Essex (see Section II).

BRANDON, THOMAS. Admitted to practise medicine 19 Jan. 1634–5. *Ibid. f. 201.*

CLARKE, ROBERT, of Barking, co. Essex, chirurgeon. Admitted on the same day. *Ibid.*

WEOLEY (WILEY in text), WILLIAM, of St Leonard's, Foster Lane, London, barber-surgeon. On a certificate from Michael Andrewes, esquire, John Warde, Nicholas Heath, and William Huckle, Masters of the Company, after examination by William Clowes, esquire, Richard Watson, esquire, Henry Blackley, and Lawrence Cotton, Masters in Surgery, dated 21 May 1636. *Ducke, f. 204.*

CRAWLEY, GEORGE, of St Gabriel's, Fenchurch Street, surgeon. Licensed after a similar certificate, and the same examiners, 20 May 1636. *Ibid.*

COPPINGER, ADAM, of St Giles without Cripplegate, London, barber-surgeon. As last two, dated 25 May 1636. *Ibid. f. 205.*

NEWTON, JOHN, literate. Admitted to practise medicine, 28 March 1636–7. See Section II. *Ibid. f. 214.*

LUSKIN, THOMAS, (no parish), chirurgeon. Admitted 2 March 1635–6. *Ibid. f. 233.*

NEWTON, JOHN. Admitted to practise medicine, 11 April 1636. *Ibid. f. 225.*

COOKE, EDWARD, of Hedingham, co. Essex, chirurgeon. Licensed 2 Oct. 1637. *Chaworth, f. 9.*

THURSTON, THOMAS, chirurgeon. Licence to practise, 2 Nov. 1637. *Ibid. f. 17.*

NIXON, RICHARD, of Brainford (?), co. Essex, chirurgeon. Licence to practise, 2 Dec. 1637.
Ibid. f. 23.

SYMEON, ROBERT, (no place), chirurgeon. Licence to practise, 4 Feb. 1637–8. *Ibid. f. 27.*

VODKA, ALEXIUS, 'Medicus' of Yorke. Certificate of conformity (see Appendix, IX), dated 12 Sept. 1639.
Ibid. f. 43.

According to Munk (*i, 193*), a 'Scotchman born'. He held an outside licence from the College of Physicians, 1627, and married a daughter of Sir George Palmer of Naburn. He was buried in St Saviour's, York, 14 May 1666. Pre-

27

sumably a son of Alexius Vodka, a Pole (*vide Munk, i, 147*). Both lived in St Saviour's parish. The elder Vodka was buried in 1644.

SUATOSSIUS, JOHN. Licence to practise medicine, dated 6 June 1639.   *Ducke, f. 57.*

WARNER, THOMAS, (no place). Licence to practise medicine, 'sub manibus in Physicis doctorum', dated 9 Sept. 1640.   *Ibid. f. 81.*

CLEVELAND, MATHEW, (no place), chirurgeon. Licence to practise, 10 Sept. 1640.   *Ibid. f. 81.*

NEWTON, SAMUEL, clerk, rector of Great Sampford, co. Essex. Licence to practise medicine, under the hands of doctors in physic, 15 Sept. 1640.   *Ibid. f. 83.*
He matriculated as sizar at St John's College, Cambridge, Lent 1620–21. B.A. 1624–5. M.A. 1628. Priest (St David's) 1658. Vicar of Great Sampford 1634–83. Buried there 12 Aug. 1683. A benefactor of his College (*Venn, Alum. Cant.*).

BATTY, THOMAS, of Uxbridge, co. Middlesex, chirurgeon. Licence to practise, Dec. 1640.   *Ibid. f. 97.*

FRYER, JOHN, of St Dunstan in the West, London, Doctor in Physic. Certificate of conformity, under the hands of Benjamin Hinton, Vicar of Hendon, co. Middlesex, and of William Turner, churchwarden there, viz. that 'he was on Sunday the fourth day of July last, present at the whole morning service and sermon in the parish church of Hendon, and did there also receive the Communion in both kinds,... of the truth whereof faith was made before us more at large. He was personally present on Sunday 9 Jan. last, at publique praiers in my chapell or oratorie at Fulham...', dated 10 Feb. 1644–5.   *Ibid. f. 104.*

WATSON, WILLIAM, citizen and barber-surgeon, (no place). On a certificate from Nicholas Heath, Henry

Boone, Masters of his Mystery, after examination by Henry Blackley, John Heydon, George Donne, and Martine Browne, Masters in Surgery, dated 19 July 1640.   *Ducke, f. 109.*

He was Master of his Company in 1657.

BOWDEN, THOMAS, barber-surgeon, (no place). Licence granted on the same date, etc., as above.   *Ibid.*

He was a Warden of his Company in 1660, Junior Warden in 1654, when he gave a cup to the company. He was in trouble in 1638, arraigned before the Court for an unsuccessful cure, and was committed to the Compter.

WORRALL, DANIEL, (no place). A licence similar to the last was granted to him on that date.   *Ibid.*

Licence to dissect an anatomy in 1648.

TURNER, ROBERT, (no place). Licensed to practise medicine, 23 March 1660 (see Section II).
                                                   Ibid. f. 123.

DEAVNISH, JOHN. Licence (in full), but see Section II.
                                                   Ibid. f. 135.

HASELOCKE, JOHN, barber-surgeon, of London. Copy of letters testimonial from John Fredericke, Alderman of London, Thomas Allen, Abraham Clerke, and Thomas Bowman, Masters of the Mystery of Barbersurgeons, after examination by Edward Arris, Henry Boone, Robert Bullocke, Charles Hamford and Laurence Loe, dated 23 April 1651, followed by the full text of a licence granted 28 May 1661.
                                                   Ibid. f. 129.

A John Haselock is said to have embalmed Oliver Cromwell. He was dead at the end of August, 1661 (*Sir Norman Moore, Hist. St Bartholomew's Hospital, ii, 316*).

DIXON, ROGER, barber-surgeon, (no place). A similar enrolment to the above.   *Ibid.*

CONEY, JOHN, citizen and barber-surgeon of London. Copy of the certificate under the hands of (blank) Turner, Thomas Bowden, John Sotherton, and Thomas Burton, Masters of the Mystery of Barber-surgeons, after examination by Henry Boone, Robert Bullocke, Thomas Allen, Nicholas Brethus, Masters in Surgery. *Ducke, f. 131.*

Perhaps identical with John Conny, Esq., Master in 1689.

HOLDITCH, SAMUEL, chirurgeon, (no place). Copy of the certificate under the hands of John Frederick, esquire, Thomas Allen, Abraham Clerke, and Thomas Bowden, after examination by the examiners. *Ibid. f. 134.*

His certificate to practise, from the Barber-Surgeons' Company, is dated 1655.

Note that in this place the following original letter is pasted into the register:

To Mr. Edward Alexander, in Doctors Commons:

Sir—All the members of our Company, as well all those who already had the Bishop of London's Licence as those who have only our Diploma, are sumon'd to attend the Bishop of London's Visitation on the 18th instant. Now Sir I thought (as to those who have our Diploma, and who I am pretty sure you cannot oblige to take your Licence,) It had been agreed between you and I, that I would send you all I could by persuasion, and that you would not endeavour to compell 'em, The Company is so alarmed at this extraordinary proceeding That if you persist in it, we must of necessity engage in a Suit at Lawe whereby to settle this point. I am Sir.

your most obedient Servant

CHAS BERNARD*

Barber's & Surgeon's Hall
  Oct. 8, 1715.

* Clerk of the Company.

ROSSINGTON, HENRY. Licence (in full), dated 23 Sept. 1662 (see Section II). *Ducke, f. 200.*

DORRINGTON, JOHN, chirurgeon, (no place). Licence in full on a certificate by the Masters of the Company, after examination by Edward Arris, Robert Bullock, Thomas Allen, and Charles Stamford, dated 29 July 1663. Signed by Richard Chaworth, the Chancellor. *Exton, f. 11.*

He presented a tankard to his Company in 1663. A John Dorrington was surgeon to the Lock in 1683 (*Sir Norman Moore, Hist. St Bartholomew's Hosp. ii, 341*).

LAYFIELD, WILLIAM, of All Hallow's, Barking, barber-surgeon. A licence similar to the last, but with the addition of John Knight as an examiner, dated 3 Aug. 1663. *Ibid.*

He was a Warden of his Company in 1686–8, and Master in 1691. In Poll-Tax, 1692/3, of St Dionis Backchurch, with wife.

CLIFFE, HENRY, chirurgeon. Licence on certificate from Thomas Lisle, esquire, Nicholas Brethus, James Farr, and Joseph Bynns the Masters of his Company, dated 22 July 1663. *Ibid. f. 12.*

SPEERE, JOHN, of St John's Zacchary, London, barber-surgeon. On a certificate of John Frederick, esquire, Thomas Allen, Abraham Clerke, and Thomas Bowden, Masters of his Company, after examination by William Kemp, Edward Arris, Henry Boone, Robert Bullack, Charles Stanford, and Laurence Loe, dated 9 Jan. 1663–4. *Ibid. f. 21.*

Perhaps John Speare, surgeon to St Bartholomew's Hosp. 1664. Died in office July 1665 (*Sir Norman Moore, Hist. St Bartholomew's Hosp. ii, 628*).

GOLD, JOHN, of St Mary's Mounthaw, chirurgeon. After the vague 'in arte predicta multorum Britorum (*sic*) laudabili testimonio', dated 9 May 1664. *Ibid. f. 26.*

31

AUSTIN, JOHN. Licensed to practise medicine, 19 Sept. 1667 (note only). *Exton, f. 47.*

CLEVELEY, JAMES, of Theydon Garnon, co. Essex. Licensed to practise medicine, 23 June 1669 (note only). *Ibid. f. 49.*

LAMBERT, JAMES. Licensed to practise medicine and surgery, 1 Nov. 1669 (note only). *Ibid. f. 49.*

GRANDEAM, JOHN. Licensed to practise chirurgery, 14 Feb. 1675–6 (note only). *Ibid. f. 74.*

LUDDINGTON, JOHN, (no particulars). Licensed 10 April 1676. *Ibid.*

RAMSEY, ARTHUR, (no place). Licensed to practise medicine and chirurgery, 19 March 1671–2.
Ibid. f. 87.

ROLFE, FRANCIS, (no place). Licensed to practise chirurgery, 10 April 1678. *Ibid. f. 157.*

GUNTER, THOMAS, (no place). Licensed to practise chirurgery, (blank) Jan. 1677–8. *Ibid. f. 157.*

SEELE, THOMAS, (no place). Licensed to practise chirurgery, 3 June 1679. *Ibid. f. 173.*

TROUTBECK, JOHN, M.D. Licensed to practise medicine, 9 March 1677–8. *Ibid.*

Perhaps M.D. Cantab. 1661. Serjeant and Surgeon to His Majesty in the northern parts. Of Bramham, Yorks, in 1665. Sent as negotiator to Monk in 1659. Served in the fleet. Died 19 July 1684, of St Martin in the Fields (*Venn, Alum. Cant.*).

BACTON, JOHN, (no place). Licensed to practise chirurgery, 20 Sept. 1680. *Ibid. 201.*

SENSKALL, JOHN, (no place). Licensed to practise chirurgery, 20 Feb. 1679–80. *Ibid. 217.*

SLADE, RICHARD, (no place). Licensed to practise chirurgery, 15 March 1679–80. *Exton, f. 220.*

BOWSER, THOMAS, (no place). Licensed to practise, 22 March 1679–80. *Ibid. f. 220.*

WARD, GEORGE, (no place). Licensed to practise medicine, 29 March 1680. *Ibid. f. 220.*

NUTTON, WILLIAM, of Epping. Licensed to practise medicine and surgery, 22 June 1680. *Ibid. f. 222.*

GOBERT, JOHN, (no place). Licensed to practise chirurgery, 12 Oct. 1681. *Ibid. f. 222.*

POULLEN, RICHARD, of Colchester. Licensed to practise chirurgery, 23 March 1682. *Ibid. f. 232.*

STANLEY, JOHN, (no place). Licensed to practise chirurgery, 20 Aug. 1683. *Ibid. f. 237.*

LASINGBY, RICHARD, of St Paul's, Covent Garden. Licensed to practise chirurgery, 25 Nov. 1685.
Ibid. f. 261.

The two books from which the rest of the names in this section are taken are still in the Archive Room of St Paul's Cathedral. *Vicar-General Reg.* 1686–1704.

GIUS, or GINS, DANIEL, of St Mary le Savoy, London, surgeon. Admitted 21 May 1686.
V.G. 1686–1704, f. 28d.

JACKSON, THOMAS, of Twittenham (*sic*), co. Middlesex, surgeon. Admitted 17 Sept. 1690. *Ibid. f. 50.*

WARWICK, CHARLES, of Staines, co. Middlesex, practitioner in medicine. Admitted 9 Dec. 1690.
Ibid.

MOORE, NATHANIEL, of Terling, co. Essex, surgeon. Admitted 22 Sept. 1691. *Ibid. f. 64.*

LUDDINGTON, JOSEPH, of Brentford, practitioner in medicine. Admitted 9 Nov. 1691. *Ibid. f. 66.*

WAYLETT, JOHN, of Southweald, co. Essex, practitioner in medicine. Admitted 10 Dec. 1694.
V.G. 1686–1704, f. 117.

DE LAGE, FRANCIS, of Kelvedon, co. Essex, surgeon. (No date) *c.* 1694. *Ibid. f. 117.*

KEARSLEY, JAMES, of Hampstead, co. Middlesex, surgeon. Admitted 2 Oct. 1695. *Ibid. f. 117.*

ANDERSON, JOHN, surgeon, of Isleworth, co. Middlesex. Admitted 16 Jan. 1694–5. *Ibid. f. 117.*

COTTON, RICHARD, of St Martin in the Fields, surgeon. Admitted 24 Dec. 1697. *Ibid. f. 138d.*

WALLIS, JOSEPH, of St James in the Fields, surgeon. Admitted 3 Nov. 1697. *Ibid. f. 137d.*

PULEAN, PETER, of St Martin in the Fields, surgeon. Admitted 18 Dec. 1697. *Ibid. f. 138d.*

PLEAHILL, WILLIAM, of St Andrew's, Holborne, surgeon. Admitted 10 Feb. 1697–8. *Ibid. f. 153.*
Warden, Barber-Surgeons' Company, 1702, 1703, 1704.

PARKYNS, THOMAS, of St Botolph's without Algate, surgeon. Admitted 11 April 1699. *Ibid. f. 155d.*

DAKINS, CHARLES, of St Brides, London, surgeon. Admitted 14 Sept. 1700. *Ibid. f. 187d.*

COLE, WILLIAM, (no locality). Admitted 8 Oct. 1700.
Ibid. f. 188.

Possibly the William Cole, Esq., Warden of the Barber-Surgeons' Company, 1722, 1725, 1726; Master, 1727.

MOOSE, RICHARD, of St Anne's, Blackfriars, London, surgeon. Admitted 10 Dec. 1700. *Ibid. f. 190.*

BARNARD, CHARLES, of St Martin, Ludgate, surgeon. Admitted 20 Jan. 1699–1700. *Ibid. f. 169.*

POPE, RICHARD, of St Leonard's, Shoreditch, surgeon. Admitted 22 Jan. 1701–2.   *V.G. 1686–1704, f. 206.*

CROSS, BENJAMIN, of St Botolph's, Colchester, surgeon. Admitted 8 Oct. 1706.   *V.G. 1705–15, f. 20.*

DUGARD, THOMAS, of St Martin in the Fields, medicine. Admitted 8 Aug. 1707.   *V.G. 1686–1704, f. 40d.*

HOLDIP, HARRY, of St Clement Danes, Middlesex, surgeon. Admitted 9 Nov. 1715.
     V.G. 1705–15, f. 186d.

ADAMS, AMBROSE, surgeon, of Kensington, co. Middlesex. Licensed 20 Oct. 1715.   *Ibid. f. 188d.*

LAYMAN, JOHN, of Braintree, co. Essex, surgeon. Admitted 26 Dec. 1715.   *Ibid. f. 191.*

BARBER, HENRY, of Nayland, co. Essex, surgeon. Admitted 25 July 1720.   *Ibid. f. 97.*

COCKE, WILLIAM, of Colchester, surgeon. Admitted 1 Sept. 1720.   *Ibid. f. 97d.*

ALDERMAN, JOHN, surgeon, Chipping Barnet, co. Herts. Admitted 1 May 1722.   *Ibid. f. 127.*

JACKSON, JOSEPH, of St Mary's, Whitechappell, practitioner in medicine. Admitted 31 Oct. 1723.
     Ibid. f. 143.

WILSON, JOSEPHUS, of Enfield, surgeon. Admitted 26 Nov. 1724.   *Ibid. f. 201.*

POND, JOHN, of London, surgeon. Admitted 30 April 1725.   *Ibid. f. 143.*

MILLINGTON, WILLIAM, of St Sepulchre, London, surgeon. Admitted 26 May 1725.   *Ibid. f. 217.*

SECTION II

Original papers preserved in the Registry of the Bishopric of London.

ABBINGTON, JOHN, surgeon, of St Andrew's, Holborn. A certificate of ability under the hands of J. Arnanding, J. Tobitt, and Hugh Baxter, surgeons, and of Thomas Manningham, rector, dated 12 Jan. 1702–3. Admitted 14 Jan. following. *V.G. 1686–1704, f. 214d.*

AIME, HENRY, surgeon, of Long-Acre in St Martins in the Fields. Certifying that he served his time with Mr Isaac Aime, late surgeon to the Queen Dowager. Under the hands of John Browne, master of anatomy and surgeon, and Ferdinando Watkins, surgeon of the hall, dated 9 Sept. 1697. Admitted 13 Sept. 1697. *Ibid. f. 136.*

Licence 16 March 1693–4 as a widower aged 28, to marry Sarah Underwood of Kensington, at St Paul's, Covent Garden (Archbp.).

ALLEN, MATHEW, surgeon, of Wapping. After apprenticeship with an able chirurgeon. Certified by Charles Ferrers, Robert Milward, John Tomkine, and William..., surgeons, and also by the curate and churchwardens, dated 25 Oct. 1697. Admitted as of Stepney, 3 Nov. 1697. *Ibid. f. 137d.*

ANSELL, THOMAS, barber-surgeon of Isleworth. Apprenticed for seven years to George Lay of New Windsor, barber-surgeon, who certifies. Dated 6 Nov. 1671. Licence granted 16 Oct. 1677 by Thomas Exton, surrogate.

ANTHONY, CHARLES. Subscribed the oath of supremacy 14 Dec. 1627.

Born 1600, of Jesus College, Cambridge. M.A. 1636. Ordained Down and Connor, 1636. Vicar of Catterick, Yorks, 1662–85. Buried there 25 June 1685.

Venn, Alum. Cant.

AYLMER, SAMUEL. Physician and chirurgeon, 'haveing practised many yeares'. Certified by Thomas Hollier, chirurgeon, and John Broun, Chirurgeon in Ordinary to the King, dated 14 Aug. 1678. Licensed by Thomas Exton, 14 Oct. following.

AYLMORE (AYLMER, *V.G.*), THEOPHILUS. Practitioner of physic and chirurgery in Chelmesford, who 'hath done great cures worthy of prayse'. Certified by Nicholas Toure, M.D., John Bastwick, *medicus*, J. Betts, M.D. Licensed by Exton, 14 Nov. 1677.

BARBER, STEPHEN, citizen of London. Certified by James Ferne, Joseph Bateman, John Locker, and Richard Lee (barber-surgeons), dated 29 June 1700.

V.G. 1686–1704, f. 190.

Will proved in the Commissary Court of London, 24 Aug. 1715. In it he mentions his brothers Michael and John, and his sisters Elizabeth and Rebecca. Admitted as of St Martin in the Vintry, 10 Dec. 1700.

BARCLAY, JOHN, of St John's, Wappin(g), chirurgeon, 'where he hath been an inhabitant for two years and hath demeaned himself as a person of an honest and sober Life'. A letter from J. Russell, rector.

He was licensed, as a bachelor, aged 42, 4 Feb. 1697–8, to marry Elizabeth Watkins, a widow, of the same age, at St Mary at Hill (Archbp.), dated 31 Jan. 1699–1700.

BARNABY, THOMAS, of Fulham, barber-surgeon. Certified by William Pearse, Francis Rolfe, Thomas Ryton, and John Batty, acting on behalf of their Company. Supported by a letter from Richard

Stevenson, the vicar, the churchwardens and 39 inhabitants. No date, but in the register Exton it is given as 22 Nov. 1676.

BARNARD, EDWARD, of Great Russell Street, surgeon. Certified by Paul Margesett, James Crafford, and Christopher Robinson, 19 Oct. 1697. Admitted as of St Giles in the Fields, 13 Nov. 1697.
V.G. 1686–1704, f. 138.
He died 23 Aug. 1737.

BARROWES, EDWARD, of Epping. Certified by Cornelius Borraeus, M.D., and John of Barrowes, chirurgeon. Sworn before Thomas Pinfold, surrogate, 20 March 1676–7.

BARTLETT, WILLIAM. Only the wrapper remains, endorsed 6 Sept. 1718. Admitted to practise medicine as of Witham, co. Essex, 22 Oct. 1715.
V.G. 1705–15, f. 185d.

BAYNHAM, WILLIAM, of St Giles in the Fields. Certified by William Cookson, M.D., John Trotter, M.D., Anthony Stamp, M.D., with a letter in support from Thomas Fettiplace, curate, John Euergan, Richard Kentish and other parishioners, dated 6 Aug. 1707. Admitted 8 Aug. following. *Ibid. f. 40d.*

BELSON, EDMUND, of Edgworth (Latin). Certificate from Anthony Colley, M.D., W. Sermon, M.D., George Vaux, licentiate, Timothy Browne, apoth., who assert that for many years past he has assiduously studied the art of medicine, dated 24 July 1673.

BENTHAM, JOSEPH, citizen and barber-surgeon. Certificate from William Layfield, John Jackson, Richard Hewet, Thomas Page, Roger Knowles, John Deane, and Thomas Gardner. Signed by C. Hargrave, Clerk of their Company, 26 May 1692. Licensed as of St Buttolph without Bishopsgate, 15 Oct. 1700.
V.G. 1686–1705, f. 189.

BERKELEY, JOHN, foreign brother of the Company of Barber-Surgeons. Signed by Sir Humphrey Edwin, Kt., 19 July 1689.

BERNARD, CHARLES, citizen and barber-surgeon. Certificate dated 7 June 1700, under the hands of Robert Leeson, John Conny, William Layfield, John King, James Pearce, Thomas Page, George Horsnell, Thomas Hobbs, Thomas Leale, Roger Knowles, and John Deane, barber-surgeons. This, perhaps the original diploma from the Company, was handed in 19 June 1700, on applying for the bishop's licence.

Charles, son of Samuel Barnard, D.D., of Croydon, was born c. 1656, apprenticed 16 Aug. 1670 to Henry Boone, serving him seven years, admitted to the freedom, 1677; chosen an assistant, 1697, an examiner in 1700 in place of T. Lichfield. Serjeant-Surgeon to Queen Anne 1702. Master of his Company 1703. Surgeon to St Bartholomew's Hosp. 1686–1711. He died at Longleat, co. Wilts, 9 Oct. 1710. At the sale of his fine library in 1711 a small book fetched £28, an unprecedented price at that time. This formed the basis of one of Budgell's contributions to the *Spectator*, No. 389.

BISSE, JAMES (of Codicote, co. Herts). Certificate from Wadham College, Oxford (Latin), dated 13 June 1697.

Son of Edward Bisse, gent., of West Ham, co. Essex, matric. at Wadham 1687, aged 17, Scholar 1689, B.A. 1691, M.A. 1693–4, B.Med. 1697, D.Med. 1701. Died at Codicote 22 Oct. 1748, aet. 80.   *Foster, Alum. Oxon.*

BOLNEST (BOULNEST), WILLIAM, of White Chapell. Certified by W. Thrasher, Med. Lic., Will. Northall, Med. Lic., and Josiah Atkynson, and Thos. Thornhill, surgeons, also a letter from John Goode, the rector, and the churchwardens of Redriffe, co. Surrey, that 'being at present an inhabitant' he deserves attestation, 14 Feb. 1673–4.

BOND, JOSIAH. Undated certificate from Roger Tocketts, Thomas Maybrigte (?), Jonah Elston, and John Best, supported by a letter from James Shaw, 'M^r of King Henry ye VII^{ts} Chappel'. Admitted as of St Clement, Middlesex, chirurgeon, 27 May 1708.
V.G. 1705–15, f. 52.

Perhaps the man of that name of St Botolph's, Aldgate, a bachelor aged 23, chir. who married Mrs Anne Keys of St George, Southwark, aged *c.* 28, at St Mary Magdalen's, Old Fish Street, 27 Oct. 1668.

BORNE, JOHN (M.D.?). Note only, 'Dr John Borne to practise the art of Medicine in St Leonard's, Shoreditch, signed Richard Chaworth, Surrogate, 10 May 1662'.

BOURSOT, JAMES, of St Martin in the Fields. Undated certificate in Latin, signed 'Derbize(?), chir., Arnaudin chir., Mercier, chir.' Admitted 21 July 1698.
V.G. 1686–1704, f. 153d.

BOXWORTH, WILLIAM, of St John's, Wapping. Certified by William Cookson, M.D., William Langham, M.D., Thomas Wilkins, M.D., supported by a letter from J. Russell, rector, John Stile and James Brightman, churchwardens, dated 12 Aug. 1707. Admitted 14 Aug. following.
V.G. 1705–15, f. 40d.

BRELHIAT, FRANCIS, of Stepney. Certificate from Deffray, Med. Dr., J. Gobert, chir., Horton, chir., dated 11 April 1692. Signed Hen. Newton, Surr. Admitted 25 April 1692.
V.G. 1686–1704, f. 66.

BRIDGES, THOMAS. Certified by William Layfield, William Babington, Jacob Babington and Richard Blundell, who state that he served his apprenticeship with Mr Will. Babington of London, surgeon, and 'is duely qualified to obtain the Bishop of London's licence to practise'. Supported by a letter from Tho. Whincop, D.D., rector of St Mary's, Abchurch, where he was a parishioner. *Fiat. Lic.*, Tho. Ayloffe, Surr. Licensed 14 Sept. 1700.

V.G. 1686–1704, f. 187d.

BROOKE, NATHANIEL, of St Martin in the Fields, chirurgeon on H.M.S. *Ye London*. A certificate of which he produced. The covering letter from Lewis Burnett, curate, 24 March 1674–5, certifies that he is 'of honest life and conversation...for ought we know or have heard to the contrary'. Sworn before Thomas Exton, Surr.

BULL, HENRY (barber-surgeon), of St John's Zacchary, London. Certified by Thomas Lichfield, John Pinke, James Wall, and Bartholomew King, barber-surgeons. He was not licensed until 16 Oct. 1700, dated 21 Feb. 1699–1700. *Ibid. f. 189.*

CAMBRIDGE, NICHOLAS, of St Gyles in the Fields. The certificate, dated 11 Feb. 1673–4, testifies to his having cured John Whetstone 'of a compound fracture in legg, as also Mary Collins, being very dangerously bitten by a mastiffe, having many lacerated wounds, as also Robert Dogley, now churchwarden of Marybone Parish, of a dangerously fractured legg'. Licence was granted 11 Feb. 1673–4 by Tho. Exton, Surr.

His will (Commissary Court) is dated 19 Sept. 1679, proved 7 July following. In it he desires to be buried in the churchyard of St Giles, leaves to his wife the household goods, to his mother Mary Cambridge 40s., to his daughter Sarah £10, and £5 for her apprenticeship, Mary his daughter executrix, with his wife Susannah, and Robert Fossett, overseers. Witnesses, Thos. Ellderge, Martha Gilley, John Todelerish.

Cambridge's certificate is signed by Nicholas Stratton and Henry Habgood, churchwardens, and by Hugh Rider, chirurgeon.

41

CARTWRIGHT, AMBROSE, of St Giles in the Fields, chirurgeon. Who exhibited a certificate from his Company, with a letter from Thomas Fettiplace, curate, Thomas Collinson and Richard Read, the churchwardens. No date is given. Signed by Hen. Newton, surr. Admitted 19 Oct. 1697.

V.G. 1686–1704, f. 137.

CHATTENERRE, JOHN (surgeon), of St Martin in the Fields. Certificate dated 11 July (? June), 1698. Signed by Bussiere, A. Derbize, and J. Arnaudinoz, surgeons. Licence dated June 15 1698. Signed J. Cooke, surr. Admitted 15 June 1697.

Ibid. f. 153.

Perhaps the John Chatenerre, chir., of St James's, Westminster, aged 31, licensed to marry Eliz. Grimmeau, a spinster, aged 22, of St Paul's, Covent Garden, 12 April 1694.

Paul Bussiere, surgeon, lived in Suffolk Street, Pall Mall.

CHESELDEN, WILLIAM, citizen and barber-surgeon. Certified by Edwin Greene, Anthony Herenden, Joseph Cousins, William Layfield, William Oades, Zacchary Gibson, Richard Harvey, Joseph Greene, Alexander Geekie, Richard Blundell, and William Loupe, of the Company of Barber-Surgeons, with a covering letter from D. Goodinge, curate of St Dunstan's in the West, and the churchwardens, who testify that he is skilled in the cure of diseases, plagues, lessions and other infirmities, dated 29 Jan. 1711–12. Admitted as of St Dunstan in the East, 19 May 1712. See *Dict. Nat. Biog.*

V.G. 1705–15, f. 122d.

CHEVELEY, JAMES, of Theydon Garnon, co. Essex, gent. Certified by Henry Tichborne, John Astell, M.D., with a covering letter from James Maggs, D.D., rector, John Gudge and William Archer, churchwardens, who say 'He is a man of sober conversation that frequents the church and is alsoe conformable to his Ma^tys govvern^t both in churche and kingdome', dated 25 June 1669. Sworn before Thomas Exton, surr.

CHOKE, JOHN, chemist, etc. 'These are to certfie that John Choke, esq., is sworne and admitted in the place of chymist in ordinary to his Matie By virtue of which place hee is to enjoy all the rights and privileges thereto belonging, his person is not to be arrested or detained without my leave, first had obteyned, nor is hee to beare any publique office nor to bee impanelled on any inquest or Jury, nor to be warned to serve at Assizes or Sessions whereby he may pretend excuses to neglect his Ma^tys service. But is to attend to the same according to his oath and duty. Wherefore I require all persons to forbeare the infringing of the privileges of the said John Choke, as they will answer the contrary at their perills. Given under my hands and seale this 11th day of July 1667, in the 19th yeare of his Maties Reigne. Signed Manchester.' (Edward Montagu, Earl of Manchester, appointed Lord Chamberlain of the Household 1 June 1660.) Granted a licence to practise medicine by Francis Hall, 11 July 1667. Endorsed John Cheke.

A notorious quack who practised in the Strand.

CLARK, JOHN, of Colchester, chirurgeon. Subscribed the oath of supremacy, 7 Nov. 1631.

CLARKE, JOHN, of Billeryck(ay), co. Essex, physician and chirurgeon. Admitted 12 Dec. 1631.

CLERKE, JOHN, of Hedingham Castle, co. Essex, apothecary and practiser in Physic in Brentwood. Certified by Chr. Jeffries, lisent., J. Chaplin, Thos. Smith, Lis., S. Dale, Licent., dated 10 Oct. 1714. Admitted 30 Sept. 1715.   *V.G. 1705–15, f. 184.*

COLLEY, ANTHONY, of St Leonard, Shoreditch. Certified by Edward Edwards, M.D., Thomas Oakes, M.D., Richard Dignan, M.D., and Will. Surman, M.D. Licensed by Thos. Exton, Surr., 1 Dec. 1669.

COO, THOMAS, of Sidney Sussex College, Cambridge. Certified by George Bowle, Med. Reg., Reuben Robinson, and Richard Reddrich, Med., Antho. Gratiano, philomed., John Hutt, Herbert Grey, Giles Aleyn, John Head, Arthur Browne, Brabazon Aylemer, Solomon Sibley, after approval by the Chancellor, in the presence of John Howgrave, 20 Dec. 1661 (Latin). Sworn before Master Smith, clerk, surrogate, 20 Jan. following.

He was admitted pensioner, aged 18, 3 May 1636, son of William Coo of Stow, co. Essex, where he was born. Educated at Maldon School. *Venn, Alum. Cant.*

CORNWALLIS, PHILIP, of Harwich, surgeon. On certificate from John..., Ab. Bincks, John Fiske, and George Hitchin, and commended by William Curtis, minister, dated 5 Sept. 1715. *V.G. 1705–15, f. 188d.*

Will, dated 29 June, proved 30 July 1729. Wife Elizabeth a third part; other parts to daughters Mary and Anne, plate to be divided amongst children; Cousin, Mr George Brook, 5 guineas. Father, the Rev. Thomas Cornwallis, and George Brook, of Allington, Suffolk, executors. *Comm. Lond. (Essex and Herts) 202 Corey.*

COTTON, RICHARD, surgeon (no locality). Certified by Jacques Wiseman, William Wood, John Browne, T. Rulean, chirurgeons, under cover of a letter from the Rev. W. Lancaster and his churchwardens, dated 21 Dec. 1697.

CROSS, BENJAMIN, of St Bottolf's, Colchester. Certified by William Dammant, John Holmested, William Nicholas, John Layman, Thomas Ireland, curate, and others, 5 Aug. 1706.

CROXTON, EDMUND. Certified by Thomas Harris, M.D., and George Impey, M.B., who say 'that he hath by his great diligence and many years studye atteyned to an eminent knowledge both in ye Theorye and Practice of Physicke'. A licence was granted, dated 10 July 1662.

CURTIS, JOHN, physician, vicar of Takeley, co. Essex. Certified by William Collyn, Thos. Heyford, Augustine Joles, Joseph Geary, and Robert Curtis, who say 'that He hath by his great diligence... many years practice and experience atteyned to much skill'. Licence granted by Richard Chaworth, Surr., dated 12 June 1662.

Perhaps pensioner at Caius College, Cambridge, where he entered 21 Jan. 1614–5, son of John Curtis, gent., of Frekenham, co. Camb. Educated at Bury. Scholar 1615–21, B.A. 1618, M.A. 1622, priest at Lincoln 1632, curate of Brandeston, co. Suffolk, of Naughton 1647, rector of Takeley, 1661, vicar of Thaxted, 1662–70.

Venn, Alum. Cant.

DABBS, JOHN, M.A., of St Giles beyond Cripplegate (physician). Certified 12 April 1665 by Jeremiah Astell, M.D., John Collop, M.D. and R. Barker.

DAKINS, CHARLES, chirurgeon. On his application he gave in the following: 'William R., William and Mary, by the grace of God, King and Queen of England, etc. To our trusty and well beloved Charles Dakins, Chyrurgeon, greeting. We do by these presents constitute and appoint you to (be) the chyrurgeon to our 2nd Regt. of our Foot guards, called the Cold Streamers, commanded by our trusty and well-beloved Colonel Thomas Talmath, You are therefore carefully and diligently to discharge your duty of chyrurgeon by doing and performing all manner of (things) thereunto belonging, and you are to observe and follow such orders and directions from time to time as you shall receive from your colonell or any other your superior officer, according to the Rules and discipline of Warr. Given att our Court at Whitehall, the first day of January 1689/90, in the first year of our Reigne. Signed SHREWSBURY'. Enclosed in a letter from Fran. Stannard, curate, dated 24 Sept. 1700.

Charles Talbot, who signs, was at the date Lord Chamberlain, created Earl of Shrewsbury 30 April 1694.

DAMMANT, WILLIAM, of Colchester. Certified 10 July 1706 by Robert Taylor, Walter Gosnold, Christopher Sparkes, and Robert Seaman. Licensed by Humphrey Henchman, surr.

V.G. 1705–15, f. 16d.

DEAVNISH, JOHN, chirurgeon, citizen and freeman of London, of St Olave, Old Jewry. Certified by Robert Bullock, Charles Stamford, William Watson, and Enoch Bostock. Admitted by the Chancellor in his chamber in the presence of W. H., notary public, dated 20 March 1660.

DE FOLLEVILLE, GEORGE, surgeon-apothecary of Chesthunt. A personal letter in French, without date, in which he states that he has been instructed in his art for three years, and has administered remedies. He implores the protection of 'your Grandeur' and leave to practise. Licence was granted 27 April 1693 by the Bishop (Henry Compton) and he was sworn before Henry Newton.

V.G. 1686–1704, f. 84.

DICKINS, AMBROSE, barber-surgeon. Certified by Gratian Bale, Edmund Green, Simon Lynch, William Layfield, Thomas Gardiner, Charles Bernard, William Oades, Zacchary Gibson, Anthony

Herenden, and Richard Harvey, dated 17 March 1709–10. Admitted 27 March 1710–11.

V.G. 1705–15, f. 84.

He was son of George Dickins, gent., of Riplington in East Meon, co. Hants. Born in 1687, apprenticed to Charles Bernard for seven years, admitted to the freedom of the Company 1709. Married his master's daughter, and succeeded Bernard as serjeant-surgeon. Elected surgeon to the Westminster Hospital 1721, and to St George's 1733, Master of his Company 1729, and died about 1747. *Young, Annals.*

DORRINGTON, RALPH, of Southminster, barber-surgeon. A letter from Robert Turner, vicar, and others, that 'he has performed very great cures as well in the parish of Southminster as in the neighbouring parishes'. Sworn 30 Oct. 1706, after exhibiting a certificate of his skill. Fees paid £1. 11s. 0d.

V.G. 1705–15, f. 21.

DOWNES or DOWNING, THOMAS, of St Mary's, Whitechapel. Letter of recommendation from William Masswell(?), curate, of Wapping, William Redding, constable, and the churchwardens, James Hall and John Welch, dated 6 April 1669. Licensed by Richard Lloyd, Surrogate, 6 Oct. following.

DRAPER, JOSHUA, bachelor of Physic, of Braintree. Certificate from W. Swallow, M.D., Al. Burnet, M.D., under cover of a letter as follows: 'Mr Butler, Mr Draper of our town, Bachelour of Physick, was promised by my Lord of London a licence at the Visitation, whenever he should send up a certificate according to law, in order to it. He hath not been unmindfull ever since but was unwilling to request a testimony of any practitioners below him, and Doctors of Physick are not so plentifull hereabouts. He had ye hand of one with whom he was joyned in consultation and because it was required to speed

47

up his certificate he hath now sent to a physician in London for his with whom he hath often been in consultation. Robert Cox, Braintree, March 22, 1664'.

Possibly the Joshua Draper, admitted a pensioner at Emmanuel College, Cambridge, 12 Aug. 1631, as of Essex, Matriculated 1631, M.B. 1638, dated 23 March 1664.
Venn, Alum. Cant.

DRINKWATER, JOHN, of New Brentford. Certified by Samuel Packer, minister, and others, and by Thomas Jackson, John Goslead(?), chir., John Rees, apothecary, 24 Aug. 1697. Licensed 10 Sept. following, by G. Cooke, Surrogate. *V.G. 1686–1704, f. 136.*

EASTGATE, EDWARD, of Poplar. Certified by Edward Layfield, Thomas Marriott, Harry Halls, John H. Porter, and many others, 1662.

ELTON, THOMAS, chirurgeon. Letter attesting his conformity. Signed Sa. Freeman, dated ...Oct. 1697. Admitted as of St Paul's, Covent Garden, 18 Oct. 1697. *Ibid. f. 137.*

EVERET, ABRAHAM, doctor of physic, of Colchester. Letter in support signed by Tho. Eyre, rector of Much-Hockesley, Marke de Pouns, rector of Wivenhoe, John Nettles, rector of Lexden, Paul Duckett, rector of St Leonard's, Richard Pulley, rector of Fordham, and Thomas Norton, that 'he is a man of pious conversation, orthodox in judgement, sound in the faith, and an obedient sonne to the Church of England', dated 18 Dec. 1661.

Everet was a student at Leyden in medicine and theology and a member of the Dutch colony in Colchester, 4 Oct. 1657, and then aged 29. He took his degree of M.D. at Leyden in 1655 (Innes-Smith).

FERNE, THOMAS, of St Clement's Lane, co. Middlesex, surgeon, and foreign brother of the barber-surgeons.

Certified by Thomas Litchfield, the Master and Ch. Hargrave, the clerk of the Company, 5 March 1699–1700. Admitted 15 Feb. 1708–9. Certified to practise medicine by Peter Gelsthorp, M.D., Thomas Lewis, Thomas Hewett, W. Everett, dated 14 Feb. 1708–9.   *V.G. 1686–1704, f. 206d.*

FINCH, THOMAS, of Much Hadham, co. Herts, physician. Certified by Peter Gelsthorp, M.D., Coll. Medicor. Lond. Soc., Tho. Lewis, Tho. Hewett, W. Everett, as 'well qualified to practise physick', 14 Feb. 1708–9.

Will, dated 30 Sept., proved 2 Nov. 1736. Daughter Sarah, wife of John Want of Hadham, bricklayer, a guinea, and her children John and Sarah, £5 each. Daughter Mary, wife of Phillip Traherne of Stansted, grocer, a guinea, and her son William, £5. Daughter Anne, messuages, etc., residuary legatee and executrix. *Comm. Lond. (Essex and Herts) 445 Andrewes.*

FIRMIN, JOHN, of Colchester, gent. Certified by Richard Morton, M.D., e Colleg. Lond., Charles Goodall, M.D., e Colleg. Lond., Jacques Wiseman, chirurgeon, Ste. West, chirurgeon, 15 Nov. 1676. Licensed by Th. Exton, Surrogate.

FLETCHER, THOMAS. Certified by Edmund Cooper, M.D., and Francis Constable, M.D. Licensed by Rich. Chaworth, Surr. ...1662.

FREEMAN, JOSEPH, of Little Waltham, chirurgeon. Certified by Benj. Chamberlaine, Licent. in Chelmsford, apothecary, Will. Swan, apothecary, in a covering letter signed by H. Thompson, the rector, the churchwardens and others, 13 April 1692. Licence granted by Henry Newton, Surr., 25 April following.   *V.G. 1686–1704, f. 66.*

FRENCH, ROBERT, chirurgeon, of St Pancras (? Soper Lane, London). Letter 'I having had some knowledge of Mr French, the bearer hereof doe suppose him to be a good chirugion and fitt to be licensed'. Signed by Elisha Coysh, M.D., with a similar letter from Wm. Savage, Med. Licent., dated 29 April 1669. *Fiat lic.* Tho. Exton, Surr.

FYGE, alias FRYE, THOMAS, physician (no place). Certified by Na. Ward, Wm. Sampson, and Lionel Lockyear, physicians. 'Mr Thomas Fyge is not only a generall learned man, but well grounded in ye rudiments of Physicke, and hath bine well discipled and seene muche practice'. Approved and sworn 3 Dec. 1661, John Williams, Surr. Endorsed Thomas Frye, in medic. stud. coram Nic. Brett Bypgeate.

GARRETT, JOHN, of Chelsey, Middlesex. Certified by R. Whiston, M.D., J. Stubbs, chirurg., Thomas Caistor, chir., Edw. Woodward, chir., John King, rector, etc., undated. Admitted 23 Dec. 1700.

V.G. 1686–1704, f. 190.

GAUDINEAU, JAMES, of St Martin in the Fields, surgeon. Certified by C. Everard, A. Ince, Wm. Munden, chir., Wm. Finch, chir., dated 14 Feb. 1675–6. Licensed by Tho. Exton, Surr.

GAY, ROBERT, of St Andrew, Holborn, citizen of London and free of the barber-surgeons. Certified by Henry Rossington, Master, John Clarke, Thomas Caistor, George Minikin, Thomas Page, George Horsnell, William Layfield, and Roger Knowles, who sign under a covering letter from Zacchary Wells, curate of St Andrew's, dated 4 Nov. 1698. Certificate dated 9 July in the same year.

Ibid. f. 16.

GEERARDS, GONSAL, of the Hague, surgeon. 'The Maister and Governors of the chirurgeon's Company att the Hague, at the request of Gonsal Geerards, our confrater or brother that the same . . . in the year

50

1658, here at the Hague hath made his proof and tryall of his art in the quality of Maister Chirurgeon, and that wee do hold and acknowledge the same for one of the brethren in the aforesaid society or hall. Therefore giveing him the power to open shopp at all times and to pracktice the art of chirurgery...att the Hague the xxixth of July 1669. Confirmed with the seale of the Companye or Brothershipp. Signed. A. de Wilde Maister, Borgoine Gouvernour, Henry Dorken hoostman' (translation dated 28 Oct. 1675). The seal is illegible.

GIDLEY, JOHN, of St Bennet Fink, London. A note that he exhibited his diploma from 'C. hall' dated 20 Dec. 1677, with a letter from Franc. Bridge, curate, Fabian Browne and Nicholas Wood, churchwardens, dated 20 Feb. 1678–9, stating that 'he hath commonly attended church'.

GILES, STEPHEN, physician. Certified by Christopher Crelle (Spinowski, M.D., of Leyden), John Groenewell, M.D. (John Groenveldt, M.D., Utrecht), John Crickton, M.D., e Coll. Med. Lond. (John Crichton, M.D., Rheims), and Sam. Munford, M.D., dated 31 March 1698.

GIRVAN, JOHN, of Childerwick (? Childerditch, co. Essex), physician. Certified by Will. Hales, physician, Th. Godfrey, M.D., Robt. Deimsell, Jo. Crichton, M.D., with a letter from Sam. Hulme, vicar, and others, dated 6 March 1707. Admitted 10 March 1707–8.   *V.G. 1705–15, f. 50.*

GLANVILL, THOMAS, of Wapping, surgeon, foreign brother of the Barber-Surgeons' Company. Sworn in the time of Roger Knowles, Master, and enrolled in the Register, with a covering letter from Nath. Resbury, rector of St Paul's, Shadwell, Robert Kyrby and Alex. Roberts, churchwardens, dated 16 Aug. 1694. Admitted as of St Paul's, Shadwell, 18 Dec. 1697. *V.G. 1686–1700, f. 138d.*

GOODIER, CHARLES, of Essex Street in St Clement Danes, surgeon. Certified by Thomas Gardiner, Roger Knowles, Francis Rolfe, and Joseph Needham, with a covering letter from J. Pride, curate, and the churchwardens, dated 21 Dec. 1697. Admitted 22 Dec. 1697. *V.G. 1696–1704, f. 138d.*

From his will (*P.C.C. Smith, 82*) dated 8 June 1706 we gather he desired to be buried in the church and had a wife, Penelope. To his three children, Penelope, Lucy, and Richard, he left £500 each. He left legacies to the daughters of his brother Francis, the children of his deceased brother Edward, Mathew Lancaster of St Andrew's, Holborn, Hester his wife, and Richard Chapman of St Clement's, an apothecary. He wishes his marriage article of 13 Aug. 1696 to be carried out and makes Lancaster and Chapman executors.

GOULD, WILLIAM, of St Stephen's next St Alban's, physician. Certified by Joseph Sone 'Theologus et Med. studiosus', Thos. Botterill, M.D., John Cotesworth, M.D., Richard Heath and Roger Nupkyn, dated 16 May 1679. Licensed by Thomas Exton, surr., 14 July 1679.

GRANT, GREGORY, of Eldam (? Elmdon, co. Essex), M.A. Certified by James Wellwood, Hans Sloane, J. Garth, Hugh Chamberlen, Fellows of the Royal College of Physicians of London, as 'fittly qualified to practise physick anywhere without the ten miles round London', dated 12 April 1712. Admitted 15 April following. *V.G. 1705–15, f. 120.*

GRAVETT, JOHN, of New Brentford, co. Middlesex, surgeon. Certified by Sam. Packer, minister, John Gisby, John Drinkwater, Robert Roberts, Thomas

Govan, chirurgeons, dated 1 Nov. 1697. Admitted
12 Nov. following.   *V.G. 1686–1704, f. 138.*

GRAY, EDMOND, Fellow of King's College, Cambridge,
physician. Certified by Charles Scarburgh, Coll.
Med. Lond. Soc. et Anat., Professor publicus, J.
Packer, Tho. Fetteplace, 'that he hath studyed and
practized Physic seven years, we judge him a person
fitting to practize publicly', dated 4 June 1662.

Admitted to King's from Eton, aged 15, 6 Aug. 1649, as
of Saffron Walden, co. Essex, Matriculated 1649, B.A.
1653, Fellow 1652–55.   *Venn, Alum. Cant.*

GREEN, EDWARD, of Christ Church, London, surgeon.
Exhibited his diploma signed by Robert Leeson,
John Conny, John King, and William Layfield,
dated 7 June 1687. Licensed 30 Sept. 1700.
                                    Ibid. f. 188.

Possibly Warden of the Barber-Surgeons' Company in
1710.

HALL, HENRY, of Deptford, co. Kent, chirurgeon. Certified Richard Holden, vicar, George Stanhope, D.D.,
lecturer, Salisbury Cade, M.D., Isaac Loader, J.
Fownes, who say that he 'hath been master chirugeon of his Maties Shipps, particilarly of a second-
rate ship, ye Rainbow, as appears by a warrant dated
1678, and thatt he hath ever since been a Practitioner
in the parish of Deptford, and hath proved himself
industrious, skillful, successfull and charitable, &
ready to assist poor seamen and souldiers in their
distress, and is also a person of entire conformity to
the Church of England', dated 10 Nov. 1699. 'I believe
this to be true. Evelyn.'

Licensed to marry, as of Deptford, a widower, aged 50,
Sarah Ireton, a spinster of St Giles in the Fields, 12 Nov.
1698, in Lincoln's Inn Chapel.

HALL, STEPHEN, of St Mary's, Whitechapel, surgeon. A foreign brother of the Company of Barber-Surgeons, wherein he was enrolled 11 May 1697. Certified by C. Hargrave, clerk of the Company, with a covering letter from Rev. Wetton, rector, and John Leave, churchwarden, dated 3 Dec. 1697.

V.G. 1686–1704, f. 138.

HARGRAVE, ABRAHAM, of St Giles without Cripplegate, London, physician. Certified by R. O. Turner, med et..., Thomas Mailson, M.D., Simon Wilson, M.D., Ja. Deane, M.D., dated 30 June 1666. Sworn before John Williams, Surr.

HARRIS, JOHN, of Lambeth Street, Whitechapel, surgeon and apothecary. Certified to have been admitted as a foreign brother to the Company of Barber-Surgeons, as of Goodmans Fields, 16 June 1692, under cover of a letter from Richard Wetton, the rector, that he is known to come constantly to Church, dated 24 Dec. 1694. Admitted 31 Jan. 1699–1700. *V.G. 1686–94, f. 177.*

HARRISON, ROBERT, B.A. (? of Kelvedon, co. Essex). Certified by John Talbot, vicar of Kelvedon, John Harrison, vicar of Burnham, John Angier, rector of Inworth, and Ben. Allen, M.B., of Braintree, dated ...1706. Licensed by Hum. Henchman, Surr. Admitted 14 July 1706. *V.G. 1705–15, f. 15d.*
Perhaps the Robert Harrison, a pensioner at Queen's College, Cambridge, 12 June 1691, B.A. 1694, who Venn supposes may have been rector of Luddenham 1713–55, and curate of Oare till his death on 1 May 1755.

HASELFOOT, ROBERT, of Harwich, surgeon. Certified by Charles Nichols, M.D., Henry Bull, and Edward Woodward, chir., dated 29 Aug. 1706, and a memorandum that he 'did serve Mr Th. Haselfoot of this towne, surgeon, deceased, as his apprentice for seven years, and hath practised the said art in this place...being surgeon to Her Majesties Pacquet Boats here'. Signed And. Smith, Thos. Phillips, churchwardens, and Thos. Langley, dated 24 Aug. 1706. Admitted to medicine and surgery, 7 Dec. 1691 and 29 Aug. 1706.

V.G. 1686–1704, f. 66; V.G. 1705–15, f. 20.

He died 12 June 1748, aged 70, and was buried at Great Dunmowe, co. Essex. The pacquet boats were used by the postal service of the time.

HAST, PHILIP, of Coggeshall, co. Essex, surgeon. Certified by James Boys, Robert Taylor, Walter Gosnold, William Dammant, and Robert Seaman, chirurgeons, dated 11 July 1706. Licensed by Hum. Henchman, Surr.   *V.G. 1705–15, f. 16.*

HAWKES, JOHN, of London, physician. Certified by Robert Johnson, John Green, Augustine Clarke, and Theo. Newman, who state that he has worked in France, Flanders and Germany for 23 years, dated 10 Aug. 1668. Licensed by Rich. Chaworth, Surr.

HILTON, JOHN, of St Giles in the Fields. Certified by John Browne, medic. et chirurgus, Surgeon in Ordinary to His Majesty, and Edward Ryse, dated 17 May 1665. Licensed by Tho. Exton, 27 May 1675.

HITCHCOX, ROBERT, of Ware, co. Herts, apothecary and chirurgeon. Certified by P. M. Sparcke, Dr. Medic. Reg., Philip Elliott, rector of Hunsdon, Ric. Waugh, vicar of Ware, as 'skilfull in the art of an apothecary, and painfull in his office of a chirugion, in the same art initiated att Chirugeon's Hall, London, and knowne by our experience to be fitt and able to practise Phisicke', dated 22 Aug. 1662.

HOLLOWAY, HENRY, of St Dunstan's in the West, surgeon. Certified by C. Dakins, Ro. Stuart, David

55

Allen, and T. Young, chirurgeons, and supported by Devereux Goodinge, curate, Th. Robinson and Wm. Freeman, churchwardens, dated 30 June 1730. Admitted 3 July 1709–10. *V.G. 1705–15, f. 72.*

HOLMESTED, JOHN, of St Mary's, Colchester. Certified by Walter Gosnold, William Dammant, J. Nicholas, Robert Seaman, Benj. Cross, John Eldred, Esq., and Ra. Kinneir, rector. No date. Admitted 8 Oct. 1706.
Ibid. f. 20d.

HUBBART, GABRIEL, of St Bottolph's without Aldgate, physician. Certified by George Wikeman, Edmund Gray, M.D., Rychard Boughton, M.D., 1 Oct. 1667. Licensed by Thos. Exton, Surr.

HUGHES, JOHN, of ... (?), surgeon. Certified by Charles Harper, Edward Harris, chir., James Bailey, chir., and Gabriell Jones, dated 25 Nov. 1675. Licensed by Ri. Raines, Surr.

JEFFREY, EDMUND, M.A., late of Peterhouse College, Cambridge. Certified by Simon Welman, Richard Blackmore, Robert Stone, and Francis Grigg, rector of Raweth, co. Essex, dated 14 July 1697. Licensed by Hen. Newton, Surr. *V.G. 1686–1704, f. 135.*
Admitted as a pensioner, aged 17, 1657, the son of a grocer at Southminster, B.A. 1661–2, M.A. 1665, ? vicar of Tolleshunt Major 1668 and of North Fambridge 1682, vicar of Boreham 1682, deprived of both 1691, (?) vicar of North Shoebury 1707–11. *Venn, Alum. Cant.*

JEFFREY, John, (?) of Whitechapel, surgeon. Certified by Robt. Baker, chir., James Bailey, chir., Gabriell Jones, chir., 4 Feb. 1675. Licensed by Thomas Exton, Surr.

KENSEY, WILLIAM, of St Dunstan's in the West, London, surgeon, after exhibiting a diploma dated 2 Aug. 1694. Certified by the minister, churchwardens and common council of the Parish, 'that he hath been an inhabitant...about fourteen years, and is a person of civill life and conversation, and hath practised all that time...with a very good and faire reputation'. Signed by John Grant, vicar, Sam. Keble and Henry Coxed, churchwardens, John Wells, deputy, John Reynolds and Charles Gretton, common council, dated 26 Feb. 1699–1700. Admitted 20 Jan. 1699–1700. *V.G. 1686–1704, f. 177.*

KENT, JOHN, of St Mary's Whyte Chapell, chirurgeon. Certified by John Hardy, chir., James Lambe, chir., Edward Edwards, chir. and John Smith, chir. Licensed by Nich. Lloyd, Surr. Dated 16 Nov. 1669.

KINGSTONE, STEPHEN, of Brentwood, chirurgeon. Certified by Nicholas Tows, M.D., John Wassten, chir., Thomas Seale, chir., dated 13 Aug. 1671. Licensed by Thos. Exton, Surr.

Will (*Arch. Essex, Hills, 264*) dated 29 March, proved 21 April 1679. Copyholds to mother, Eliz. Dore; after her death to John and Thos., sons of Thos. Satch, of Goldanger, Essex, drugger. Christopher Francis, Mary his wife, and Mary his daughter, £10 each. Brother-in-law, Thos. Satch, £10. Anne Greithead of Brentwood and Anne, her daughter, £10 each. Residue to mother, executrix.

KNIGHT, JOHN, of Castle Hedingham, co. Essex, chirurgeon. Admitted according to the statute 15 Dec. 1634.

KNOWLES, ROGER, of St Brides, London, citizen and barber-surgeon. Letter from Henry Dove, D.D., vicar, Henry Perris and David Lumsden, churchwardens, that as 'one of our parishioners he doth orderly frequent the said parish church. Received the Sacrament...on Easter Day last, 28 Jan. 1678–9', dated 14 Feb. following. Licensed by Thos. Exton.

Warden of the Barber-Surgeons 1689–90, Master 1693.

LAMB, JAMES, of Norton Folgate in St Leonard's, Shore-
ditch, physician and surgeon. Certified by John
Ellys, M.A. and Edward Gelsthorpe, fellows of Caius
College, Cambridge, John Mote, M.B., late fellow
of St John's, Titus Oates, B.A., anatomist of St John
the Divine, 'quondam alumnus', late student of
Gonville and Caius, dated 1 Nov. 1669. Licensed by
Thomas Exton, Surr. (Latin).

Ellys, Gelsthorpe, and Mote were reputable but Oates had
no such degree. See *Dict. Nat. Biog.*

LANGLEY, SAMUEL, of Harwich, surgeon. Certified by
Charles Nichols, M.D., Henry Bull and Edward
Woodward, chirurgeons, under cover of a letter from
Richard Tye, mayor, Thomas Langley, Justis',
Andrew Smith and Thomas Philips, chirurgeons,
dated 29 Aug. 1706.   *V.G. 1705–15, f. 20.*

LAPWORTH, JOHN, of St James's, Clerkenwell. Certified
by John Ricqburgh, surgeon, G. Bustre and Edward
Jennyngs, chirurgeons, under cover of a letter from
Deverel Pead, minister, Thos. Elford and Richard
Flower, churchwardens, dated 24 Sept. 1711.
               V.G. 24 Sept. 1711, f. 113.

LA ROCHE, JOHN ANTHONY, of St Martin in the
Fields, surgeon. Certified by J. Arnauding and Dec.
Baluds (?), chirurgeons, dated 9 June 1697. Ad-
mitted 14 June 1697.   *V.G. 1686–1704, f. 135.*

LATHRUP, or LATTRAUP, ROBERT, of Stepney,
physician. Certified by George Thomason, M.D.,
Robert Cooper, M.D., John Askew, M.D., 'candi-
datus', Nicholas Sudell, M.D., 'licent', dated 15
Jan. 1666–7. Licensed by Richard Chaworth, Surr.,
26 Jan. 1666, 'On which day appeared before mee
Robert Lattrauf and subscribed to ye act of Uniformity renouncing ye Solemn League and Covenant
before mee Richard Chaworth'.

LAWLESS, NICHOLAS, (no place or date). He 'served a terme with Jn Browne, a surgeon in the army, and had experience in ye art of surgery both at home and abroad'. Signed by ... Rolfe, John Browne, Samuel Stubbes, and Hugh Ryder, under cover of a letter from Samuel Prat, D.D., minister of the Savoy and Robert Nicholson, churchwarden. Admitted as of St Mary le Savoy, 29 Oct. 1697.   *V.G. 1686–1704, f. 137d.*

LE NEVE, ROBERT, physician. Certified by Matthew Brooke, D.D., Amos Rideing, B.D., Tho. Reeve, B.D., Ri. Dukeson, B.D., and John Southwell, M.D., his instructor, who say that he 'is the sonne of Jeffrey le Neve, Doctor in Physick, was educated by his said father and by him diligently instructed in that noble science, under whome he had practice soe long as he lived. But after the death of his said father betooke himselfe to Doctor John Southwell and practised with him, and by his owne industry and helpes aforesaid (being alsoe the inheritour of all his said father's bookes, notes, and phisicall observations), with the knowledge and experience of ten years practice, and many varityes and rare receptions which he hath, is well approoved of by those that knowe him, and because he hath wrought many excellent cures, it is much desired by many that hee may be admitted to practise and administer physick in his owne name, hee being alsoe of an honest life, and ciuill, sober, sweet conversation, and allwayes very carefull to do all the good that he can for the health of his patients', dated 13 May 1662. Licensed by Richard Chaworth, Surr.

LITEGOLD (LIFEGOLD, *V.G.*), JAMES, at Dorniff, a French refugee, of Rochford, co. Essex, surgeon. Certified by Pierre Daual, chir., Daniel Cooper, surgeon, J. Cailleau, chir., Daniel Delasar, chir., dated 28 Aug. 1706.   *V.G. 1705–15, f. 20.*

MASTERS, GEORGE, of St James's, Westminster, surgeon. Enclosing a certificate from the Company of Barber-Surgeons, on his appointment 'to bee chirugion's mate, John Yate being Master Chirugion, on His Maties Shipp, the Charles Gally', signed by Ch. Hargrave, Tho. Gardiner, and Tho. Caister; and another of November 1699, 'that the bearer hearoff George Masters, is Fetley Qualified to practise surgery', signed by John Williams, surgeon, and Ferdinando Watkins, under cover of a letter from Will. Wake, rector, John Riley and Ben. Turbevil, churchwardens, dated 8 Feb. 1699. Admitted 9 Nov. 1699.   *V.G. 1686–1704, f. 168.*

MEALE, ROBERT, of St John's Zacchary, citizen and freeman of the Barber-Surgeons. Certified by Sir Nathaniel Herne, Henry Johnson, Richard Powell, William Pierce, Edward Arris, John Knight, Richard Wiseman, Ralph ..., Thomas Hollier, James Pierse, and William Markham, after examination on 29 Dec. 1674, dated 11 Jan. following.

MERCIER, MICHEL, a Frenchman, surgeon. A letter in French from C. J. Lamothe, one of the ministers of the French church, Savoy, directed to Mons. le Docteur Haley, rector of St Giles in the Fields, to assure him that Mercier is a good Protestant, under a letter from the said rector and his churchwardens, Thomas Collinson and Richard Read, dated 2 July 1697. Licensed 5 Oct. following.

Ibid. f. 137.

MILLS, JOHN, surgeon, of St Clement Danes, and formerly in the Royal Navy. Certified by George Rolfe, Nicholas Lawless, Thomas Elton, and Stephen Hall of the Barber-Surgeons' Company, 21 May 1704, under cover of a letter from John Giffard, curate, John Thompson and George Jenkins, churchwardens. Licensed by Henry Newton, Surr., 31 May 1704. *V.G. 1686–1704, f. 218d.*

Probably the John Mills appointed surgeon's mate on H.M.S. *Dover*, March 1705–6. *Adm. N.B. no. 2960.*

MONEY, THOMAS, of Ware, chirurgeon. Letter from the rector, Richard Waugh, and others, asserting that 'he hath effected severall cures on divers persons', dated 31 Oct. 1670. Licensed by Thos. Exton, Surr., 3 Nov. 1670.

MONTALLIER, MATURIN, physician, (no place). Certified by James Hinton, ...Forrest, M.D., Ludovicus Molinaeus, M.D., B. Mayerius, B.M., 15 April 1669. Licensed by Tho. Exton, Surr.

MORDEN, WILLIAM, of Stepney, physician. Certified by William Freeman, Med., John Langford, M.D., Christopher Woodhouse, Med., to practise in the city and seven miles round, 21 June 1669. 'This could not passe by reason of the parties insufficiencie.'

MOUNSEY, JONATHAN, (no place). Certified by Edmund Page, Thomas Denny, James Wasse, and George Molins, who assert that he had served seven years' apprenticeship to an eminent surgeon. Dated 22 Nov. 1700. *V.G. 1686–1704, f. 189d.*

NEW, WILLIAM, of St Paul's, Shadwell, chirurgeon. 'London, these are to certify that ye Masters or Governors of ye Mistery or Comminalty of Barbers and Chirurgions of London, have appointed William New, Master Chirurgeon of their Maties Shipp the Ossery, now fitted out to sea, and he is ordered to prepare himselfe for ye service with all convenient speed, and for soe doeing this shall be the warrant'. Signed and sealed 6 Jan. 1691, Ch. Hargrave, Barbers' and Chirurgeons' Hall (original warrant upon parchment). In a covering letter from George Constable, Lecturer of St Paul's, Shadwell,

Edward Lloyd and William Bowin, chirurgeons. Admitted 20 Oct. 1697. *V.G. 1686–1704, f. 137d.*

NEWEL, JOHN, of Harwich, physician and chirurgeon. A letter from Edward Alexander, Esq., of Harwich, directed to Capt. Grey. 'The bearer hereof Mr Newel, being recommended to us for an able surgeon, and one whose character and ability y^e are wel acquainted with, he having been imploy'd in the same quality in one of the Pacquet Boats dureing the late war, in which service he behav'd himself very wel. we do hereby acquaint y^o that we have appointed him surgeon to y^r Boat, and am glad to hear he is a person very acceptable to you.' Signed R. Cotton, Tho. Frankland, Gen. Post Office, 15 May 1702, and the following: 'Sept. 2 1715, Register. The bearer hereof Mr John Newel, my parishioner, comes to wait on you according to your summons, in order to take out his licence for the Practice of Physick and Chirurgery, He is a person of known reputation, approved skill and experience in that art. But as to any fresh certificate from graduate Doctors it cannot be had in these parts, there being not any between this and Colchester (Signed) Wm Curtis, Minister'.

Will, 22 Jan. 1751, leaving all to wife, Hannah. *Comm. Lond.* (*Essex and Herts*) *407, Goodwin.*

NEWMAN, THOMAS, surgeon, of (?). Certified by Abraham Sherwell, chir., Charles Bell, surgeon, Jo. Lee, surgeon, under cover of a letter from Ric. Hollingworth, minister, and his churchwardens, and Rich. Rowe, chir., dated 20 Jan. 1699–1700.

NEWTON, JOHN, *Medicus Studiosus.* Admitted to practise, having subscribed the three prescribed articles, before 'me' freely and 'ex animo', dated 11 April 1636.

A John Newton was licensed to practise medicine 1612–13.
Venn, Alum. Cant.

NORMAN, THOMAS, of St Giles in the Fields, chirurgeon. Attestation signed by Wm. Hagley, rector, .Tho. Collinson and Rich. Read, churchwardens, 16 Oct. 1697. 'I have made enquiry...and have been informed by Mr Cooper, one of my assistants, that the said Mr Norman is a Protestant.' Admitted 15 Nov. 1697. *V.G. 1686–1704, f. 138.*

PAGE, PHILIP, of Chesthunt, co. Herts, surgeon. Certificate that he served his apprenticeship with Thomas Barber, surgeon, late of Jewin Street in St Giles's, Cripplegate. Signed by Gratian Bale, Richard Bateman, chir., Jo. Bateman, chir., and John Webb, chir., with a covering letter from R. Chapman and the churchwardens, dated 19 July 1707. Admitted 17 June 1707. *V.G. 1705–15, f. 37d.*

PAINE, JON', of St James's, Westminster, chirurgeon. Certified by Robert Peirse and Cornelius Beton, chirurgeons, Jacques Wiseman and Edward Woodward, surgeons, under cover of a letter from William Wake, rector, and the churchwardens, dated 23 Oct. 1697. Admitted 29 Oct. following.
V.G. 1686–1704, f. 137d.

PAINE, JOHN, surgeon, R.N. Certified by William Pleahill and Zachariah Gibson, governors, Charles Bernard and Richard Greene, examiners, and found fully qualified to serve as surgeon's mate on any of H.M. ships of war, 18 Jan. 1704–5. Admitted 9 Jan. 1716–17.

He was granted certificates 18 Jan. 1704–5 and 14 Nov. 1710. Mate on H.M.S. *Berwick,* then H.M.S. *Burlington,* March 1709; H.M.S. *Union,* March 1710–11; on the *Queenborough,* Aug. 1711; the *Burford,* March 1715. With these papers is the following letter dated 14 Aug. 1711, 'that last October (I being then fixed in my business at Dublin) I condescended to leave my place of abode to act

63

as Surgeon's Mate to the Queenborough, owing to the Surgeon's illness' (signed Thomas Drummond, who asks for his discharge). *Adm. N.B. no. 2961.*

PARKYNS, THOMAS, of St Botolph's, Aldgate, surgeon. Certified by Archibald Clifford, chir., and Thomas Caistor, chir., Thomas Neale and Henry Batchelor, under cover of a letter from Adam Angus, clark (*sic*), and the churchwardens, dated 11 April 1699. Licensed by Henry Newton, Surr.

PETERS, CHARLES, of St Martin in the Fields, surgeon. Certified by Jeremiah Bowden, John Prestman, chir., Sonnybanke Ghyles, who state that 'he hathe under God done severall cures in and about London', dated 22 Oct. 1674. Licensed by Thos. Pinfold, Surr.

POPE, RICHARD, of St Leonard's, Shoreditch, surgeon. Certified by William Adams, surgeon, John Clifton, surgeon, Nicholas Baxter and William Smithson, surgeons, Thomas Caister, chirurgeon, and Thomas Lyfe, surgeon, dated 22 Jan. 1701/2. Licensed by Henry Newton, Surr.

PORTER, BENEDICT, physician and surgeon. 'Under the command of his Excellency Edward Lord Herbert, Earle of Glamorgan, Generall of his late Maties Forces in South Wales. I, Thomas Cardiff, Colonell of a Regiment of Foot, do hereby certifie that the bearer hereof, Benedict Porter, Physician, hath served in my regiment as Physitian and Surgeon for the space of five years, in all wch time he behaved himself honestly and faithfully in discharge of his employment as aforesaid and also as a soldier upon all occasion of service and commands in the time of the late unhappy warres, in his late Maties Service, of moste glorious memory. and neuer deserted the performance of his duty to his King and country.' Dated 23 Feb. 17th Charles (1664–5). Signed. Accompanied by an attestation by Theophilus (Field), Bishop of St David's, written on parchment. Licensed by Richard Chaworth, Surr.

PRATT, THOMAS, of St James's, Duke Place, chirurgeon. Who exhibited his diploma as a foreign brother of his Company, dated 5 April 1687. Licensed 14 Oct. 1700. *V.G. 1686–1704, f. 189.*

PRESTON, WILLIAM, of St Buttolph's, Bishopsgate, physician. Under an attestation signed by B. Goodridge, Med. Licent. and a number of others, apparently patients, who will testify on oath that 'he is a man well affected to the present government and having been a practitioner in Phisick for above the space of six yeeres', dated ...1662.

PRICE, HUGH, of Chipping Barnet, physician. Certified by Thomas Alvey and Daniel Cox, M.D.s, dated 19 Oct. 1693. Licensed by Henry Newton, Surr.

RIDEOUT, GEORGE, of St Paul's, Shadwell, surgeon. Certified by John Tenison and Thomas Reuben, chirurgeons, 26 March 1673. Licensed by Michael Lloyd, Surr., 2 April following.

ROBJERT (ROBIENT, *V.G.*), JOHN, of All Saints, Malden, co. Essex, chirurgeon. Certified by Richard Strutt and John Long, surgeons, and J. Bowes, M.D., dated 20 July 1706. Licensed by John Johnson, Surr., 26 July 1706. *V.G. 1705–15, f. 16.*

Will dated 24 April, proved 4 July 1713. Messuage in All Saints parish to son James and silver watch, six spoons, and buckles. Residue to daughter Susannah. Executor, brother-in-law, Mr Cornelius Begard. *Comm. Lond. (Essex and Herts) 336 Backhouse.*

RODON, JOHN, of Harwich, chirurgeon. 'Harwich, Essex. We whose names are here underwritten do certify that there being no Physician in all this country nearer than Ipswich or Colchester, Mr John Rodin Chirugeon, has been oblidg'd to administer Physick to many people of all sorts and has done it with a great deal of skill and success.' (Signed) H. de Luzancy, vicar of Dovercourt and Harwich, Edmund Seaborne, rector of Oakley parva, Henry Cole, rector of Oakley magna, Robert Riche, vicar of Ramsey, Francis Upton and J. Beaufort, '*fiat Lic.*' Together with a commission from the Bishop directed to H. de Luzancy and Riche, empowering them to take the oath of allegiance, etc., dated 23 July 1697. Together with Rodon's subscription to the King, the Book of Common Prayer, and the 39 articles. Sealed with an oval seal *ad causas*, viz. the coat of arms of the See impaling Barry of eight argent and gules as many martlets in orle sable. A crescent for difference for Thomas Chaworth. Legend 'SIGILL: VICAR: IN SPI: ET VIC: GENERAL'. Admitted 8 July 1697.

V.G. 1686–1704, f. 136.

ROOKES, NICHOLAS, of Shadwell, physician, after practising in Hamburg. Certified by Robert Pratt and John Allinus, *medic.*, Charles Wilcox and John Mathewes, dated 26 June 1670. Licensed by Thomas Exton, Surr.

ROSE, JOHN, of Felstead, co. Essex. Certified by Robert Sherwood and Thomas Jacob, chirurgeons, 13 Feb. 1695–6, under cover of a letter from Benjamin Smyth, clerk, and William Child, churchwarden, dated as above. Licensed by Henry Newton, Surr. Admitted 13 Feb. 1695–6. *Ibid. f. 119.*

ROSSINGTON, HENRY, barber-surgeon. Certified by Charles Stamford, Master, Ralphe Thicknes, John Sotherton, Wardens, Thomas Hollier and Henry Cleare, 28 March 1660. Application dated 23 Sept. 1662.

Master of his Company in 1695.

66

ROUSE, JOHN, of St James's, Westminster, surgeon. He 'served seaven yeares apprenticeshipp to Paul Margett, of St Paul's Covent Garden, Surgeon to H.M. Royall Regiment of Horse Guards, and hath been out of his time three yeares last past, and practised for himself'. (Signed) John Browne, master of anatomy, of London, Joseph Vallis, surgeon, William Rome, curate.

ROWGHT, WILLIAM, of St Leonard's, Colchester. Certified by John Holmsted, John Hone, and Charles Wensloe, chirurgeons, with the churchwardens and others. No date. Admitted 20 Oct. 1697 and 29 Aug. 1706.

V.G. 1686–1704, f. 137d; V.G. 1705–15, f. 20.

Will dated 20 Oct. 1734, proved 1 Jan. 1740–41. Freeholds in St Leonard's parish to wife Elizabeth, while sole, then to son John, then son William. To wife household goods, stock of coals, 'my swan loyter and two-thirds of the Hopewell loyter', and shares in any other vessells or sloops. Wife executrix. *Comm. Lond. (Essex and Herts) 341 Bull.*

RULIAU, PETER, surgeon. Certificate from John Dubourdieu, minister of ye Savoy, that 'he is a member of his congregation and a French protestant, according to the discipline and ceremonies of ye Church of England and that he is of good reputation amongst us for his true and christian behaviour', dated London, Xber 18, 1697. (Signed by) Dubourdier. A certificate of his ability is enclosed signed by Philip Rose, Dr of physic, L. Laisne, surgeon, M. Derbald(?), chirurgeon.

SAFFOLD, THOMAS, physician, (no place). Certified by Nicholas Barbon, 'de Coll. Lond.', Henry Crawford, Richard Stone, Lic. Med., John Langford, Med.

Licent., W. Thrasher, M.L., John Hawkes, M., dated 4 Sept. 1674. Licensed by Tho. Exton, Surr.

Well-known charlatan. Born *c.* 1640. Died May, 1691. He was succeeded by the notorious John Case. Will (*P.C.C. 89, Vere*). Thomas Saffold, Licensed physitian and citizen and weaver of London. To be buried in St Martin, Ludgate, where I now live. To brother, James Saffold, of St Laurence, Tillingham, Essex all such sums as are due from him and £20; and to Wm., Thos. and James, his sons, £10, to put them out to trades. To Mary, their sister, £10 when married or 21. Executrix to 'well cloath my said two nephews and either to keepe them or send them home to their father as she shall think fitt'. To Friend, Mr Alex. Reade, a gold ringe; Servant Thos. Britch £3, and his wages. To Ralph Low and Mary, his wife, £3 each; Joseph James, 10*s.*; Thos. Bingham, 5*s.*; Joseph Munk, 1*s.*; God-daughter Sarah Rust, £5.; Mary Low, 10*s.* Poor of St Martin's, 4*d.* Residue to wife, Prudence. Wit. Edwd. Roberts, Wm. Barratt, Thos. Taylor. Proved 27 May 1691, by Prudence. Commission, 22 May 1695, to James Saffold, brother, to administer upon the death of Prudence Eaglestone, alias Saffold.

SAVAGE, WILLIAM, physician, (no place). Certified as licensed to practise by J. Elliarsere, Pract. Medic., J. Howton, Med. Reg. Ord., dated 16 April 1662.

SCOFIELD, JOHN, of Uxbridge, physician (?). Certified by Joseph Clerke, Charles Vermuyden, dated 10 May 1665. Licensed by Henry Fauconberg, 2 Oct. 1677.

SEAMAN, PAUL, B.A. Emmanuel College, Cambridge, Colchester. Certified by Sir Edward Alston, President, and Baldwin Hamey, George Ent, and John Micklewait, examiners to the Royal College of Physicians. Licensed by R. Chaworth, Surr., dated 20 April 1664.

He was admitted a pensioner at Emmanuel 24 April 1646, as of Suffolk, Extra-Licentiate R. Coll. Phy., 22 April 1664. *Venn, Alum. Cant.*

SEAMAN, ROBERT, of Colchester, surgeon. Certified by Robert Taylor, Walter Gosnold, William Dammant, Ch. Sparke, dated 10 July 1710. Licensed by Hum. Henchman, Surr. (Possibly son of the above.) Admitted 10 July 1706.   *V.G. 1705–15, f. 16.*

SHAW, THOMAS, barber-surgeon. Certified by Thomas Sargent, Henry Boon, and Robert Bullock, 11 June 1662. Approved by 'My Ld. Bp. himself at the motion of Mr Joseph Sheldon', 13 Jan. 1662–3.

Perhaps of St Botolph's, Bishopsgate, citizen and barber-surgeon. Licensed as a widower, aged 50, to marry Sarah Mearer, widow, on 5 Feb. 1665–6.

SMITH, GEORGE, of All Saints, Barking, chirurgeon. Who exhibited a diploma signed by Thomas Gardner, George Minnikin, Thomas Litchfield, and John Puck, barber-surgeons, dated 24 Feb. 1697–8. Admitted 19 Oct. 1700.   *V.G. 1686–1704, f. 189d.*

SPARKE, THOMAS, of Harwich, surgeon. Certified by Robert Taylor, Walter Gisnold, William Dammant, and Robert Seaman, surgeon, dated 10 July 1706. Licensed by Humph. Henchman, Surr.
          V.G. 1705–15, f. 16.

Will, 23 April, proved 11 May 1716. Leaves his messuages to wife Hannah, with remainder to Thomas Spark Seaman, son of Robert Seaman of Colchester, chirurgeon. To kinsman Robert Seaman, 5s. and to Mr Jacob Bury of Harwich a guinea, a brasse pistol and an Indian lance. Wife executrix.   *Comm. Lond. (Essex and Herts) 29 Bawtree.*

STARR, JOSIAH, of St Martin in the Fields, physician. Certified by Charles Morton, M.D., Oliver Horsman, M.D., and Joseph Palmer, M.D., 19 Oct. 1699. Admitted 20 Oct. following.   *V.G. 1686–1704, f. 168.*

STEVENS, SAMUEL, of the Diocese of London, chirurgeon. Subscription to the oath of Supremacy, 4 Oct. 1627.

STEWART, WILLIAM, of Winslow, co. Bucks, practitioner in physic. Letter stating that he had been in practice about 12 years and was 7 years with Mr Wm. Reynolds at Great Shelford in Cambs. Signed by Samuel Box, vicar and many others. Licensed ...1663.

STOCKTON, THOMAS, of Little All Hallows, London, physician. Certified by Richard Jackson (Librarian of Sion College), John Tomlinson, M.D., and R. Turner, M.D., dated 26 June 1661, on which date he was sworn before the chancellor.

STRUTT, EDWARD, of Chipping Ongar, co. Essex, surgeon. Certified by John Dobie, Medic., Richard Strutt, surg., Benjamin Reynolds and John Johnson, surgeons (undated). Admitted 16 July 1706.
V.G. 1705–15, f. 16.

STRUTT, RICHARD, of Chelmsford, gent., physician and surgeon. 'Educated and practised as a surgeon for these thirty years last past,...a skilfull person and fittly qualifyed to practise Physick.' (Signed) Peter Gelsthorpe, M.D. Coll. Lond. Soc., Ja. Drake, M.D., Coll. Med. Lond., Wm. Cocke, M.D., dated 2 Nov. 1705. Admitted 14 Nov. 1705.   *Ibid. f. 11.*

THORNHILL, THOMAS, of St Leonard's, Shoreditch, chirurgeon. Certified by Ambrose Atfield, D.D., Christopher Finney, curate, Thomas Hollier, Joseph Atkinson and Thomas Parker (?), chirurgeons, dated 20 Jan. 1673–4.

TONGUE, HENRY, barber-surgeon, (no place). Certified by Sir Nathaniel Herne, Henry Johnson, Richard Powell, and William Pierce ('concordat cum originale'), ...Jones, Wm. Deely, dated 11 Jan. 1674–5. Licensed by Thos. Exton, Surr.

TOTON, JOHN, of Stepney, chirurgeon (?). Certified by Arnaud Finch (?), ...Brelhiat, chir., 19 April 1692. Licensed by Henry Newton, Surr.

TURNER, Daniel, of St Botolph's, Bishopsgate, barber-surgeon. Who exhibited a diploma signed by Thomas Lichfield, Master, James Wall, John Pucke, and Bartholomew King, barber-surgeons, dated 12 June 1700. Admitted 15 Oct. 1700.

V.G. 1686–1700, f. 189.

'Intending to become a Collegiate physician he applied for his discharge from the Freedom and Livery of the Company,' 16 Aug. 1711. *Vide* Munk, *Roll of the Royal College of Physicians*, Vol. 2, p. 35.

TURNER, ROBERT, physician (?), (no place). Certified by Richard Jackson (Librarian of Sion College), and John Mulillobon, M.D., undated. Licensed 23 March 1660–61, by Dr Chaworth, Surr., in the presence of Richard Thompson and of William Angier, notary public.

TYREMAN, WILLIAM, chirurgeon. Certified by John Slingh, John Battey, Thomas Poole, Roger Locke, chirurgeons, and William Salmons, Dr, 6 April 1670, who declare him 'to bee a very honest civill person and very knowing and expert in his practice; that hee was at sea under Sᵣ Jeremie Smith, where and in other places hee hath given signall testimony of his integrity and skill'. Licensed by Thos. Exton, Surr.

VALLIS, JOSEPH, barber-surgeon, of St James's, Westminster. Admitted a foreign brother of the Barber-Surgeons' Company, sworn in the time of Sir Humphrey Edwin, entered in the register 13 Aug. 1689, C. Hargrave, clerk, under cover of a letter from Wm. Wake, Rector, John Payne and Humphrey Dudson, chirurgeons.

VAUGHAN, JAMES, of Epping, chirurgeon. Letter signed by John Shepherd, curate, and others, who say 'he is a verie able chirurgeon and hath done many good cures', dated 1 Nov. 1673. Licensed by Tho. Exton, Surr.

VERE, THOMAS, of St Clement Danes, surgeon (?). Certified by George Strutt, M.B., Roger Knowles, Abraham Showell, John Tatham, G. (blank) and Ri. Genyns, surgeons, dated 19 Dec. 1705. Admitted 21 Dec. 1705. *V.G. 1705–15, f. 11d.*

WAKERING, GILBERT. Subscribed the Oath of Supremacy 17 Dec. 1631.

WARD, JAMES, chirurgeon. Certified by Oliuer Upsalle, M.D., Nich. Sudell, Licent. Licensed after subscription to 'ye act of Uniformity, renouncing ye Solemn League and Covenant' before Richard Chaworth, 25 Jan. 1666–7. Francis Hall, Surr.

Possibly the James Ward, of Stepney, widower, aged about 50, chir., licensed to marry Mary Ridley, a widow of St Botolph's, Bishopsgate, at St Leonard's, East Cheape, 23 May 1666.

WARWICKE, RALPH, of Stanes (*sic*), physician. Certified by Jo. Butler, Ed. Holte, Med., Joshua Butler, Med., Jer. Whitaker, Med., 12 Oct. 1677, as a 'person expert in the science and faculty of phisick for neere twenty yeares, whose experience wee have often seene with good successe in many difficult cures... and is a true lover of the Church of England'. Licensed by Thomas Exton, 12 Feb. 1677–8.

WHADCOCKE, CHARLES, surgeon, and Freeman of the Company of Barbers and Surgeons of London. Certified by Charles Bernard, William Pleahill, Thos. Page, Wm. Layfield, Jas. Wall, Zachary Gibson, Edward Green, Richard Harvey, Christopher Tal-

man, and Richard Blundell, dated 14 Aug. 1704.
Admitted as of St Margaret Moses, London, 10 Nov.
1715. *V.G. 1705–15, f. 186d.*
Possibly of Bread Street, where Mr Whadcocke, surgeon,
died 17 March 1733.

WHITFIELD, THOMAS, of Staines, chirurgeon. Certified
3 March 1691 as having served as apprentice to Mr
Green, chirurgeon to Christ's Hospital. Signed by
Charles Bernard and Edward Greene, chirurgeons,
under cover of a letter from Roger Davies, vicar,
dated 3 March 1691–2. *V.G. 1686–1704, f. 166.*

WHITFORD, HENRY, of St Martin in the Fields, surgeon. Certified by Charles Peter, Christopher
Robinson, Thomas Vivian and Thomas Hollier,
dated 20 July 1679, under cover of a letter from
William Hodges, minister of St Anne's, Westminster,
and the churchwardens, dated 20 Dec. 1697. Admitted 22 Dec. 1694. *Ibid. f. 138d.*

WILLCOX, CHARLES. 'Late Master of the Pesthouse
belonginge to the Tower Hamlettes, now Chirurgeon
to his Maties Royal Garrison in the Tower of London.
Certified by Robert Pratt Dr in Phisique and Philo,
Ben. Porter, chimest, Joh. Stacy, chemest, George
Pope, practitioner in physick in White-Chappell,
Lionel Lockyer, Phisi. Licen., Licensed 29 April 1699
by Peter Lane Surrogate in Stepney, before whom
he took the Oath of Allegiance.'

WILLIAMS, JOHN, chirurgeon. 'A person conformable
to the Church of England.' Signed Sa. Freeman.
Endorsed Oct. 1697. Admitted as of St Paul's, Covent
Garden, 18 Oct. 1697. *Ibid. f. 137.*

WILLIAMS, THOMAS, surgeon, of St James's, Westminster. Certified by Ch. Hargrave, 31 July 1690,

as 'found qualified and appointed chirurgeon's mate, George Beale being Master Chirurgeon, on H.M. Shipp *Winsore Castle*', under cover of a letter from William Rome, curate, and James Thatcher, church-warden, dated 23 Aug. 1697. Admitted 5 Oct. following. *V.G. 1686–1704, f. 137.*

WILLIAMS, WILLIAM, physician. Certified by Paul Chamberlaine, Peter Dormer, William Starling, Robert Chamberlaine, Oliver Upsall, all M.D.s, and R. Barker, licentiate, dated 3 Feb. 1663–4.

WINTLE, RICHARD, of St Martin in the Fields, late of the Royal Navy, chirurgeon. Signed by W. Hall, Jn. Browne, S. Stubbes, dated 10 July 1697. Admitted 10 Aug. following. *Ibid. f. 136.*

WROTH, THOMAS, of St Leonard's, Shoreditch, physi-cian. Certified by Edward Birchworth, Philip Peers, Thomas Oakes, and William Sermon, all doctors of medicine, dated 26 Oct. 1669. Licensed by Thomas Exton, surrogate.

YONGE, WILLIAM, of Great Warley, co. Essex, physician. Letters testimonial signed by Edward Freeman, Coll., Reginald Carew, George Weldon, rector of Great Warley, William Pretty, Coll., Joseph An-drews, M.A., dated 18 Nov. 1662. Endorsed *ars med.*

APPENDIX OF DOCUMENTS

I

1529. Johannes Johnson parochie Sancti Clementis extra barras novi templi Londinensis, presentatus fuit Reverendo patri Domino Londinensis episcopo, in palacosa Londinensis, per M. Edwardum Fynche et Arthurum Malachias, in mediciniis doctores, Robertum Beverley, Thomam Gybson, Johannem Mownford, et Thomam Powtyng, gardianos artis vel Mistere Cirurgicorum, etc. assistentia Edwardi Classehend, Baldewyni Kyrkeby, Johannis Taller, et Xroferi Dixson, cirurgorum, alias admissus tanquam expertus et habilis ad occupandum et exercendum artem cirurgicam, Quem die, etc.

Foxford, f. 203.

II

Die Veneris ix die Augusti anno 1555, in quadam galleria sive perambulatorio superiori in palacio episcopali Londinensis, coram Reverendo patre Edmundo, Londinensis episcopo, in presentia mei Roberti Johnson, notarii publici, et Registarii, etc. Comparuerunt personaliter, prenominati, Thomas Vycary, Georgius Holland, et Georgius Geen, et certificarunt et affirmaverunt prenominatos Thomam Skoos, et alios, in suprascripta scedula nominatos, diligenter examinasse, admississe, etc. Quare Dominus, ad eorum instanter, decrevit literas testimoniales inde fieri et sigillari, iuxta statutum etc. cuilibet dictorum examinatorum et admissorum tradendi.

Croke, f. 201.

III. *A grant by the Chancellor*

Octavo die Februarii 1562, in domo Magistri Huycke, Vicarii generalis, etc. ac coram eum in presentia mei Petri Johnson, Registarii, etc., Dicto die presentata et exhibita fuit quadam schedula per Georgium Hollande, Richardum Ferrys, Georgium Gynne et Thomam Gale, examinatores, etc. Ad cujus relationem et commendationem, Reverendo Patri Domino Edmundo Londinensis Episcopo, quosdam Patricium Sele et Johannem Willoughbye, clericum, per eum admisse fuerunt, ad practicandum, etc. ut emanavit literas testimoniales et sub sigillo Reverendi Patris, etc.   *Huicke, f. 72.*

IV. *A more formal grant before the Chancellor*

Vicesimo sexto Martii 1580, coram Venerabili viro Magistro Edwardo Stanhope, legum doctore, officiali principali, etc. in camera sua, etc. in presentia Willielmi Blackwell, notarii, etc. comparuerunt propter Willielmum Clovey, civem et barbitonsorum Londinensis, et Willelmum Eden, clericum Misterii Barbitonsorum et Chirurgorum et ex parte Willielmi Bovee, Willielmi Crowe, et Thomae Birde, Magistrorum seu Gubernatorum ejusdem Misterii, et quadam litteram eorundem manuscripte, signatas et certificandas ejusdem Willielmi Clowes fuisse examinatum de praxi et experientia sua in arte chirurgicae per Robertum Muddesley, Johannem Field, Willielmum Bovie, et Johannem Yates, examinatores in ea parte speciales, etc. et per eos fuisse approbatum, etc. Unde prestiti primitus predictum Clowes jurato super emitat Regie Majestati, etc. Dominus ad eius petitionem admisit ipsum dictum Willielmum Clowes ad exercendum officium chirurgi, etc. et desuper dedit ei litteras testimoniales in scriptis de data predicta.   *Hamond, f. 196.*

V. *Form of admission of chirurgeon in English*

To all christen people to whome these presents shall come, John, by the providence of God Bishoppe of London, sendeth greatinge in our Lorde God everlastinge. Whereas in avoydinge dyvers and grevous hurtes and jeopardies, whiche in the Realme of Englande daylie happen by the presumptious unpunished boldnes of uncunninge chirurgeons. It was in the tyme of the famous raigne of king Henrie the eighte, wholesomelie and politiqglie enacted, ordeyned, and established, that it shall not be leafull to enie parson within the realme, to occupie or exercise the science or arte of chirurgerie, except they were firste examined and admitted by certain parsons to whome that power and aucthoritie by the said statute and acte were committed. We therefore, to whome the same aucthoritie by the said ordinance is given and committed within the cittye of London, and seaven miles in circuite abowte the same, callinge unto us fower experts, parsons in the facultie of chirurgerie accordinge to the teanour of the said statute, that is to saie Master Leonard Coxe, Richard Wood, William Borne, and George Denham, chirurgions, by our predecessors Bishoppes of London aforetyme admitted to practize the science or arte of chirurgerie, by the said arte have diligentlie examined, Hughe Lingen of the parishe of St Buttolphes withoute Algate in London, of oure diocese and jurisdiction, Barbour and Chirurgeon, and have fownde him the same Hughe Lingen, righte hable and sufficiente, to occupie and exercise the said facultie and science of chirurgerie, and as one hable and sufficiente thereunto, we have approved and admitted him, and by these presents wee doe approve and admitt him, beinge first sworne upon the holie Evangelistes before the righte worshipful Master Edward Stanhope, Doctore of the Civill Lawes, our Chancellour, to the supremacie of the Queene's moste excellente Majestie. In witnes whereof unto these presentes we have sette the seale of

77

our said Chancellour, which we use in this behalfe,
Yeoven att London, the syx and twentieth daie of
Februarie in the yeere of our lorde God, after the com-
putacioun of the Churche of Englande, one thousand
fyve hundreth eightie eighte, and in the twelfe yeere of
oure consecracioun.   *Stanhope, i, 257.*

VI

Edmundus providentia divina Norwicensis Episcopus,
dilecto nobis in Christo Johanni Croppe de Norwico,
salutem gratiam et benedictionem. Cum ex fide digna
relatione acceperimus te in Arte Chirurgie per non modi-
cum tempus versatum fuisse multisque de salute et sanitate
corporis vere desperatis (deo omnipotente administrante)
subvenisse et sanasse Necnon in arte predicta multorum
peritorum laudabili testimonio pro experientia, fidelitate,
diligentia, et industria tuis circa curas susceperis peri-
genda in hujusmodi arte chirurgie merito recommenda-
tum et ad practicandum igiter et exercendum dictam
artem chirurgie in et per Diocesam et civitatem nostras
Norwicensis ex causis predictis et aliis nos in hac parte
iuste moventibus quantum nobis per Statutam hujus in-
cliti Regni Anglie liceat et non aliter neque alio modo te
admittimus et approbamus. Tibique licentiam et facul-
tatem in hac parte tenore presentium quamdiu te bene
et laudabiliter gesseris benigne concedimus et elargimur.
In cujus Rei Testimonium Sigillum Officii Vicarii nostri
in spiritualibus generalis quo in hac parte utimur presentibus apponi fecimus. Dat. decimo sexto die mensis
Augusti anno dni Millesimo Quingentesimo Septuagesimo
septimo et nostre translationis anno secundo. Richardus
Skynner, Registrarius.

To all christen people to whome theise presents shall
come, John by the providence of God Bushopp of London,
sendeth greetinge in our Lord God everlastinge. Whereas
in avoyding of divers and grevous hurtes and jeopardies

78

which within the realme of England daylye happen by the presumptuous unpunished boldnes of uncunninge chirurgions Ytt was in the tyme of the famous Reigne of King Henrye the eighte wholesomelye and pollitickelye enacted and ordeyned and established, That yt sholde not be lawfull for any person within this Realme of England, to occupye or exercise the Scyence or arte of chyrurgerye, excepte they weare first examined and admitted by certayne persons, to whome that power and authoritie by the sayd Statute and Acte is committed. We therefore to whome the sayd Aucthoritie by the said Ordinaunce is given and committed within the Cittye of London and Seaven myles in circuit abowte the same, havinge received sufficient Testimonye from the Reverend Father in God the Lord Bushopp of Norwiche, under his seale, where John Cropp dwelleth, of the knowledge skyll and approved practize of the sayd John Croppe nowe of the Cittye of London, in the Scyence and arte of chirurgerye to be right able sufficient and skylfull to occupye and exercise the sayd facultye and scyence of chirurgerye. And is one hable and sufficient thereunto, wee have approved and admitted him the sayd John Cropp, and by these presents wee do approve and admitt him, so farr as by the lawes and Statutes of this Realme wee are authorized so to do (being first sworne upon the holye Evangelistes) before the righte Worshipfull Master Edwarde Stanhope, doctor of the Ciuill lawes and Chauncelor, to the supremacye of the Queen's most excellent Maiestie. In witness wheareof unto these presents, wee have putte ye Seale of our sayd Chauncelor, which wee use in this behalfe. Yeaven at London the firste day of Februarye, in the yeare of Our Lord God after the Computation of the Church of Englande one thousand five hundreth and nynetie, And in the fowerteenth yeare of our consecration. Will. Blakwell deputatus.   *Stanhope, ii, 20.*

VII

Richardus permissione divina, Londinensis Episcopus, dilecto nobis in Christo Petro Lambert clerico, in artibus Magistro, curato Ecclesie Parochialis de Braxted Magna in Com. Essex in nostrae Londinensis Diocesie et jurisdictionis, Salutem in domino. Ad exercendum et practicandum artem medicinalem et medicandi in et per Diocesim nostram London. Civitate London. duntaxas excepta ac ad dandum et ministrandum medicinas et medicamenta salubria ac consilium medicinale omnibus et singulis subditis domine nostre Regine infra diocesim nostram London. eadem recipere volentibus. Tibi de cuius fidelitate et conscientie puritate plurum confidimus in hac parte. Ac de scientia et experientia medicinalibus et in arte medicandi fide dignorum testimonio plenius informamur, quantum in nobis est, et de jure ac Statuti hujus Regni Anglie possumus et non aliterque alio modo, licenciam concedimus spiritualem durante nostro bene placito ac dummodo honeste prudenter et vere te gesseris in hac parte, per presentes prestito prius per te iuramento supremitatis Regine Majestatis. In cuius rei testimonium Sigillum vicarii nostri in spiritualibus generalis et officialii principalis, in et per totam civitatem et diocesim London. quo in hac parte utimur presentibus apponi fecimus. Datum tertio die mensis Decembris, anno domini millesimo quingentesimo nonagesimo septimo, et nostre consecrationis anno primo.   *Stanhope, iv. f. 10.*

VIII

John permissione divina Londinensis episcopus, nobis in Christo Roberto Luskin de Harwich in comitatu Essex. nostrae Londinensis diocesie, et jurisdictionis, Salutem in domino, etc.

Exercendum et practicandum artem chirurgicam et

artem medicandi, in et per totam diocesim et jurisdic-
tionem nostram Londinensis. (Civitate Londinensis et
locis statuto in hac parte prohibitis dumtaxat exceptis),
iuxta tenorem statutorum hujus Regni Anglie ea parte
editorum ac ad dandum et ministrandum medicinas et
medicamenta salubria ac consilium medicinale, omnibus
et singulis domini nostri Regis infra diocesim nostram
Londinensis, (exceptis ut supra), eadem recipere volentibus sibi de cuius fidelitate et conscientie puritate plurimum
concedimus in hac parte Ac de scientia et experientia
chirurgicis et medicinalibus et in arte sanandi et
medicandi chirurgica et medicinale ex...fide dignorum
et in artibus predictis peritorum testimonio in hac parte
requisito plenius informamur quantum in nobis est, et de
jure, ac statutis hujus Regni Anglie possimus et nobis
licet et non aliter neque alio modo durante se bene-
placito et dummodo honeste et prudenter te gesseris in
hac parte, licentiam concedimus specialem per presentes
prestito per te prius sponte iuramento supremitatis Regie
Majestatis sui hac parte edita et prescripta. In cuius rei
testimonium, sigillum Vicarii nostri in spiritualibus
Generalis, quo in hac parte utimur, presentibus apponi
fecimus. Dat. Londini (blank) die mensis Novembris
anno domini 1618 et nostro consecrationis anno octavo.

V. G. Marten, i, f. 102.

IX. *Certificate upon the conformity of
Alexius Vodka, medicus*

William, by the providence of God, Bishop of London,
Lord High Treasurer of England To all christian people
to whome theis presentes shall come sendeth Greeting in
our Lord God everlasting.

Know ye that Alexius Vodka of the City of Yorke,
Practitioner in Physicke, upon the day of the date of
these presentes was personally present before me; and

being as he then alledged indicted and convicted for Recusancy, and for not repaireing to Church to heare divine Service and Sermons, according to the lawes of this Realme in that case provided, did willingly submitt in his due obedience to the King's most excellent Majestie. And in further Testimony of his Conformitie he was present upon the day of the date of theis presentes at publique praiers in my Chappell scituate within my Mannor of Fulham in the County of Middx. from the beginning to the ending therof, orderly and decentlie demeaneing himself, as well in my presence, as in the presence of divers others there assembled, and hath further faithfully promised and professed and under writeing with his own hand acknowledged, to continue his conformitie in diligent and usuall repaireing to publique praiers and receiving the Sacrament of the Lords Supper according to the rightes and ceremonies of the Church of England, as by Dutie and the said Lawes he is bound to performe. And moreover the said Alexius Vodka willinglie and of his owne accord took his othes of the Kinges Supremacy and of his Obedience and allegiance to his Sacred Majestie according to the Statute in that case provided willingly and utterly renouncing all obstinacie, and faithfully promiseing to continue in obedience to his Majestie and the Church of England. In witness whereof I have hereto set my hand and seale episcopalle, the Twelfth day of September in the Yeare of our Lord God one Thousand sixe hundred and Thirtie nine and in the sixth yeare of my consecration.

Chaworth, f. 43.

X. *Certificate of Sion College*

Reverendissimo in Christo patri Gilberto, providentia divina episcopo Londinensis, salutem in domino sempiternam. Cum presentium Exhibitor Robertus Turner

generosus, pro Quadremio in Collegio Sionensi Rei
Medicae studiosus sua industria in eadem scientia multum profecerit, et multis hujusce Regni subditis languore
Laborantibus suppetias tulerit: ad desiderium dicti
Roberti Liberum istius artis quam (ut opinor) exorte callet
exercituum, cupientis, vestrae dominatione testatum eo,
prefatum Robertum in facultate praedicta tales fecisse
progressus, quibus per multis morbo et vario dolore inde
oboriente perituris opem tulerit In cujus Rei Testimonium hasce literas nostrae dominationi offerendas
humillime subscripsi.

Richardus Jackson, Artium Magister, et Sionensis
Bibliothecae consutus Inquisitor.

Iterum testatur Jo. Mulillobon. M.D.

Admissus coram Doctore Chaworth vicesimo tertio die
mensis Martii Anno Domini 1660. in presentia Ricardo
Thompson et Willielmi Angier Notarii Publici.

XI. *Certificate of Royal College of Physicians*

Notum cupimus omnibus, id quos id scire attinet, nos
Edwardum Alston, Equitem Auratum, Medicinae
doctorem, et presidentem Collegii Medicorum Londinen-
sium, una cum Balduino Hameii Georgio Ent et Joanne
Micklewait ejusdem Collegii examinasse probum virum
Paulum Seaman pronuper in Collegii Emanuelis Canta-
brigiae in artibus Baccalaurium, nunc vero Colcestriae
in comitatu Essexiae medicinam practicandum eundemque dignum iudicasse, qui ad medicinae practicandum
per Angliam admittatur; modo id ne fiat intra civitatem
hanc ejusque circum vicina poemeria easque porro lege,
ac conditione ut in arduis negotiis aliis aliquem peritum
medicum in consilium advocet; eundemque praeterea
privilegiis omnibus secundum Regni statutum debitis
ornavimus. In cujus rei fidem ac testimonium Tabulas
hasce sigillo nostri munitus ipsi concessimus nominaque

subscriptionis vicesimo secundo die Aprilis anno Domini millesimo sexcentesimo sexagesimo quarto

> Edwardus Alston
> Balduinus Hameii
> Geo: Ent, Registerius
> Johannes Micklethwaite.

Concedet licentiam

> R. C.

XII. *Midwifery* *

Examinatio et admissio obstetricum xviii° die mensis Septembris A° Domini millesimo quingentesimo xxvi° coram Magistro Wharton officiali in presentia mei Johannis Irlond.

Uxor (blank) Conway parochie Sancte Marie Magdalene in piscaria exhibuit litteras examinacionis et admissionis facere sub sigillo Domini Fitjames (Richard Fitzjames, bishop, 1506–22) nuper episcopi Londinensis.

Elizabethe Bekett uxor Johannis Bekett parochie Sancti Sepulchri, exhibuit litteras ejusdem Domini Episcopi.

Ansia Fynche, parochie de White Chappel admissa et jurata et dixit non habuit litteras quare Dominus assignavit ad probandum per ii testes in crastino vel citra die dominica proxima sequentes advenineiis(?) Dicto die compuerunt Josatam Aviliam et uxorem Aumer Bateman et Johanna Freman parochie predicta in testes, que dixerunt quod ante fuerunt tempore admissionis fine ad x annos elapsos ut modo recolent coram Magistro Hedd ad hunc officium, etc. Et demandaverunt litteras auctoritate episcopi moderni.

Joanna Williamson vidua parochie Sancte Swythenii dicta assignavit ad subeundam examinam pro sua ad-

---

* Lovers of Tristram Shandy will remember that Yorick, the parson of the village in which Shandy Hall was situated, 'cheerfully paid the fees for the ordinary's licence himself, amounting in the whole, to the sum of eighteen shillings and fourpence'; for the 'thin, upright, motherly, notable, good old body of a midwife', who assisted at the birth of Tristram.

missione et quod adducat secum dua obstetrices citra...
proximo et casu quo non erit admissa quod non exerceat
post illum diem sub pena excommunicationis.*

Alicia Banaster vidua parochie Omnium Sanctorum
Stanynges cui Dominus assignaverit prout assignatus est
Johanne Williamson proximo precedenti.

XIII. *Certificate granted to a midwife*

Secundo die mensis Julii anno 1557, domo Magistri
Thomas Darbyshere, Vicarii Generalis, etc. et coram et
in presentia mei Roberti Johnson, Registrarii, etc. com-
paruit dicta Margeria Munte (de Bursted magna), et
secum intro duxit Agnetem Harrys, Dorotheam Harrys,
et Agnetem Clercke, Et tunc dictus Magister Darbyshire
examinavit eandem Margeriam secrete de eius practicia,
etc. et experientia et praxi in dicta arte prefata. Mulieres
introducte et per dictum vicarium generalem examinate et
interrogate publicum et laudabilem proferebant testimonium et eandem Johannam tanquam discretam idoneam
et expertam ad officium hujusmodi exercendum multum
laudabunt et commendabant quam quidem Margeriam
Munte sic laudatam et commendatam dictus Magister
Darbyshere admisit in obstetricem in et per comitatu
Essexiae, primoris per eam iuramento corporali, etc. et
fideliter et indifferenter exercendo dictum officium, etc.
faciendo observando et per implendo iuxta tenorem soliti
iuramenti, etc. Licet per eum prestitit et decrevit sibi
literas testimoniales.   *Croke, f. 302.*

* This is valuable as showing the procedure in the cases of these
women who were in danger of excommunication if they practised
without the leave and imprimatur of the court.

XIV. *Certificate in English to a midwife*

These are to certifie y^t Margaret Corney, widow, by Practice Midwife, is a person loyall to his Ma'tie, a dutifull and obedient daughter of ye Church of England her mother, of knowne and experienced abilitye in her profession of Midwifery, as by sufficient testimony of many persons she hath delivered, will be made good and hath beene an inhabitant of the parish of St Peter Paul's Wharfe forty yeares.

(Signed) Joh. Williams Rector Ecclesie Sⁱ Petri iuxta ripam Paulinam Dat. 11. Novemb: 1661.

James Medlicott⎱
John Boddy ⎰ Churchwardens.

Elizabeth Hales, midwife, aged 83.

Mary Scredin her marke, midwife, aged 80.

Testes p'dict. examinat' et Jurat. ac Margareta Corney Jurat, Coram Magistro Jo. Wms (John Williams), surro (gato).

*A table of Vicars-General of the Diocese of
London, 1530–1715*

Richard Foxford, D.C.L., 1530.
Nicholas Wotton, LL.D., 1533.
John Storye, LL.D., 1539.
John Crooke, LL.D., 1543.
William Clyff, LL.D., 1547.
Henry Harvey, LL.D., 1550.
Griffin Leyson, LL.D., 1552.
Nicholas Harpesfeld, 1554.
John Wymsley, 1554.
Thomas Darbishire, D.C.L., 1556.
*Thomas Hunwicke, D.C.L., 1559.
John Hamond, LL.D., 1570.
Sir Edward Stanhope, LL.D., 1577.
Sir Thomas Crompton, D.C.L., 1607.
Thomas Edwards, D.C.L., 1608.
Sir Henry Marten, D.C.L., 1618.
Arthur Ducke, D.C.L., 1624.
Sir Richard Chaworth, D.C.L., 1660.
Sir Thomas Exton, D.C.L., 1668.
Sir Henry Newton, D.C.L., 1688.
Humphrey Henchman, D.C.L., 1715.

From the list in the Bishop's Registry.

* Huycke in text.

INDEX NOMINUM

The names of the Licencees are marked with an asterisk.

Apoth. = Apothecary.
B.S. = Barber-Surgeon.
Md.   = Midwife.

P.   = Physician.
P. & S. = Physician and Surgeon.
S.   = Surgeon.

*Abbington, Jn., S., 36
*Abbis, Thos., P. & S., 22
(Abbot), Geo., Bp., 21
*Adams, Amb., 35
— Wm., S., 64
*Aime, Hy., S., 36
— Isaac, 36
Alcocke, Nic., S., 15
*Alderman, N., 35
Alexander, Edw., 62; letter to, 30
Aleyn, Giles, 44
Allen, Ben., P., 54
— David, S., 55
*— Math., S., 36
*— Ra., 25
*— Thos., B.S., 23, 29, 30, 31
Allinus, Jn., M.D., 66
Alston, Sir Edw., 68, 83–4
*Altofte, Rbt., S., 23
Alvey, Thos., M.D., 65
Alyeffe, Jn., S., 13–14
*Anderson, Jn., 34
Andrewes, Mich., B.S., 27
— Jos., M.A., 74
*Angir, Jn., S., 13; R. of Inworth, 54
Angus, Ad., Clk., 64
Annatt, Thos., S., 18
*Ansell, Thos., B.S., 36
*Anthony, Ch., V. of Catterick, 21, 37
Arnauding, J., S., 36, 40, 42, 58
*Arris, Edw., S., 23, 29, 31, 60

Arris, Jasp., S., 23
Askew, Jn., M.D., 58
Astell, Jn., M.D., 42
— Jeremiah, 45
Atfield, Amb., D.D., 70
Atkinson, Jos., S., 70
Atkynson, Josiah, S., 39
Atmer, Lew., 19
*Austin, Jn., P., 32
Aylemer, Brab., 44
Aylmer, Jn., Bp. of London, 78, 80
*— Sam., P. & S., 37
*Aylmore, Theo., P. & S., 37
Ayloffe, Thos., 41

Babington, Jacob, B.S., 40
— Wm., B.S., 40
*Bactere, Jn., Clk., 15
*Bacton, Jn., S., 32
Bailey, Jas., S., 56
Baker, Alex., S., 23–5
— Rbt., S., 56
Baldewyne, Hy., S., 13
Bale, Grat., B.S., 46, 63
Balthropp, Rbt., 16
Baluds (?), Dec., S., 58
Banaster, Alice, 85
(Bancroft), Ric., Bp., 80
Bankes, Thos., S., 17
*Barber, Hy., 35
*— Steph., S., 37
— Thos., S., 63
Barbon, Nic., M.D., 67

88

*Barclay, Jn., 37
Barker, Alex., S., 22
— R., P., 45, 74
*Barnaby, Thos., B.S., 37
*Barnard, Ch., 34
*— Edw., S., 38
*— Rbt., 21
*Barrowes, Edw., S., 38
*Bartlett, Wm., 38
Bastwick, Jn., P., 37
Batchelor, Hy., S., 64
Bateman, Jn., S., 63
— Jos., B.S., 37
— Joyce, Md., 84
— Ric., S., 63
Batty, Jn., B.S., 37, 71
*— Thos., S., 28
Baxter, Hugh, S., 36
— Nic., S., 64
Bayley, Thos., S., 16
*Baynham, Wm., 38
Beale, Geo., S., 74
Begard, Corn., 65
Bekett, Eliz., w. of Jn., Md., 84
Bell, Ch., S., 62
*Belson, Edm., P., 38
*Bennet, Wm., S., 24
*Bentham, Jos., B.S., 38
*Berkeley, Jn., B.S., 39
*Bernard, Ch., B.S., 39, 46, 47, 63, 72
— Clerk of the Company, letter of, 30
— Sam., D.D., 39
Best, Jn., 40
Beton, Corn., S., 63
Betts, J., P., 37
Beverley, Rbt., S., 12, 75
Bincks, Abr., 44
Birchworth, Edw., M.D., 74
Birde, Thos., B.S., 16, 76
*Bisse, Jas., 39
Blackley, Hy., B.S., 23–4, 27–8
Blackmore, Ric., 56
Blundell, Ric., B.S., 40, 42, 73
*Blundye, Alard, S., 15

*Bond, Jos., S., 40
(Bonner), Edm., Bp., 75
Boone, Hy., B.S., 29–31, 69
*Borne, Jn., M.D., 40
— Wm., S., 18, 77
Borraeus, Corn., P., 38
*Bostocke, Enoch, S., 25, 46
Botterill, Thos., M.D., 52
Boughton, Ric., M.D., 56
*Boulnest, Wm., P., 39
*Boursot, Jas., S., 40
Bovie (Bovee), Wm., B.S., 16–19, 76
Bowden, Jer., 64
*— Thos., B.S., 29–31
Bowes, J., M.D., 65
*Bowin (Bowyne), Jn., S., 14
— Wm., S., 62
Bowle, Geo., M.D., 44
*Bowling, Xph., 13
Bowman, Thos., B.S., 29
*Bowser, Thos., S., 33
*Boxworth, Wm., P., 40
Boys, Jas., S., 55
*Brandon, Thos., P., 26
Brethiat (?), Fra., S., 40, 71
Brethus, Nic., B.S., 30–1
*Bridges, Thos., S., 40
Britch, Thos., 68
Brooke, Geo., 44
— Math., D.D., 59
*— Nath., S., 41
Browne, Arth., 44
— Jn., P. & S., 55
— Jn., S., 36–7, 44, 59, 67, 74
— Mart., B.S., 29
— Tim., Apoth., 38
*Bull, Hy., B.S., 41, 54, 58
*Bullock, Rbt., B.S., 24, 30–1, 46, 69
*Burgis, Jn., S., 17, 20
Burnet, Al., M.D., 47
— Lewis, Clk., 41
Burton, Thos., B.S., 30
Bussiere, P., S., 42

Dale, S., P., 43
*Dammant, Wm., S., 44, 46, 55–6, 69
Daval, Pierre, S., 59
Deane, Jn., B.S., 38–9
— Jas., M.D., 54
*Deavnish, Jn., S., 29, 46
Deely, Wm., 70
Deffrey, —(?), M.D., 40
*De Foleville, Geo., S., 46
Deimsell, Rbt., 51
*De Lage, Fra., 34
Delasar, Dan., S., 59
Denham, Geo., S., 18, 76–7
Denny, Thos., S., 61
Derbize (?), —(?), S., 40–2
*Dickins, Amb., B.S., 46
— Geo., 47
Dignan, Ric., M.D., 44
*Dixon, Rog., B.S., 29
Dixson, Xph., S., 12, 75
Donne, Geo., B.S., 29
Dorken, Hy., 51
Dormer, Pet., M.D., 74
*Dorrington, Jn., S., 31
*— Ra., B.S., 47
Doughton, Arth., 23, 25
Dove, Hy., D.D., 57
*Downes (Downing), Thos., 47
Drake, Jas., M.D., 70
*Draper, Josh., P., 47
*Drinkwater, Jn., 48
Drummond, Thos., 64
Dubourdieu, Jn., Min. of Savoy, 67
Duckett, Pa., R. of St Leonard's, 48
Dudson, Humph., 71
*Dugard, Thos., 35
Dunn, Geo., S., 24

*Eastgate, Edw., 48
*Eaton, Hy., S., 22
Eden, Wm., B.S., 16, 76
Edwards, Edw., M.D., 44; S., 57
Edwin, Sir Humph., B.S., 39, 71

Elderge, Thos., 41
Elliarsere, J., P., 68
Elliott, Ph., R. of Hunsdon, 55
Ellys, Jn., M.A., 58
Elston, Jonah, 40
*Elton, Thos., B.S., 48, 60
Enderby, Jn., S., 14
Ent, Geo., P., 68
Evelyn, Jn., 11, 53
Everard, C., 50
*Everet, Abr., M.D., 48
— W., 49
Eyre, Thos., R. of Much-Hockesley, 48

Farr, Jas., B.S., 31
Fauconberg, Hy., 68
Ferne, Jas., B.S., 37
*— Thos., B.S., 48
Ferrers, Ch., 36
Ferris, Ric., S., 14–16, 75
Fettiplace, Thos., 38, 42, 53
*Field, Jn., S., 15–16, 76
— Theoph., Bp. of St David's, 65
Finch, Ansia, Md., 84
— Edw., M.D., 12, 75
*— Thos., S., 49
— Wm., S., 50
Finney, Xph., Cur., 70
*Firmin, Jn., P. & S., 49
*Fisher, Edw., S., 22
Fiske, Jn., S., 44
(Fitzjames), Ric., Bp. of London, 84
*Fletcher, Thos., P., 49
*Foster, Wm., B.S., 20
Fownes, J., 53
Frederick, Xph., S., 20
— Jn., alderman of London, 29, 31
Freeman, Edw., P., 74
— Joan, 84
*— Jn., S., 49
— Sam., 48, 73
— Wm., P., 61

*French, Rbt., S., 49
*Frye (Fyge), Thos., P., 50
*Fryer, Jn., M.D., 28

Gale, Thos., B.S., 14, 16, 76
*— Wm., S., 17–19
Gardiner, Thos., B.S., 46, 52, 60, 69
*Garland, Ra., S., 12
*Garret, Jn., 50
Garth, J., M.D., 52
*Gaudineau, Jas., S., 50
*Gay, Rbt., B.S., 50
Geary, Jos., 45
Geekie, Alex., B.S., 42
Geen (Gynne), Geo., B.S., 14–16, 75–6
*Geerards, Gonsal, S., 50
Gelsthorpe, Edw., M.D., 58
— Pet., M.D., 49, 70
Genyns, Ric., S., 72
Ghyles, Sonnyb., 64
Gibson, Thos., B.S., 12, 13, 75
— Zacc., B.S., 42, 46, 63, 72
*Gidley, Jn., 51
Giffard, Jn., Clk., 60
*Giles, Steph., P., 51
*Gins, Dan., S., 33
*Girvan, Jn., P., 51
Gisby, Jn., 52
*Glainvill, Thos., B.S., 51
*Gobert, Jn., S., 33, 40
Godfrey, Thos., M.D., 51
*Gold, Jn., S., 31
Goodall, Ch., M.D., 49
Goode, Jn., R. of Redriffe, 39
*Goodier, Ch., S., 52
Goodinge, Dev., Clk., 42, 56
Goodowrus, Wm., S., 19
Goodridge, B., P., 65
Goslead (?), Jn., S., 48
Gosnold, Walt., S., 55–6, 69
*Gould, Wm., P., 52
Govan, Thos., 53
*Grandeam, Jn., S., 32
*Grant, Greg., M.A., 52

Grant, Jn., 57
Gratiano, Ant., P., 44
*Gravett, Jn., S., 52
Gray, Edm., M.D., 56
*Graye, Sam., 17
*Green, Edm., 43, 46, 53
— Edw., 72
— Jn., P., 55
— Jos., B.S., 43
— Ric., B.S., 63
Grey, Capt., 62
— Hbt., 44
*Griffith, Maur., S., 26.
Grigg, Fr., R. of Raworth, 56
Groenewell, Jn., M.D., 51
*Gunter, Thos., S., 32

Hagley, Wm., R. of St Giles in the Fields, 63
Hales, Wm., P., 51
Haley (? Hagley), Ric., R. of St Giles in the Fields, 60
*Hall, Hy., S., 48, 53
*— Steph., B.S., 54, 60
— W., S., 74
Hamey, Baldw., M.D., 68, 83–4
Hamford, Ch., B.S., 29
Hardy, Jn., S., 57
*Hargrave, Abr., P., 54
— C., Clk., 38, 49, 60–1, 71, 73
— Xph., B.S., 49–54
Harper, Ch., S., 56
Harris, Agn., Md., 85
— Dor., Md., 85
— Edw., S., 56
*— Jn., B.S., 54
— Thos., M.D., 45
Harrison, Jn., V. of Barnham, 54
*— Rbt., B.A., 54
Harvey, Ric., B.S., 72
*Haselfoot, Rbt., S., 54
— Thos., S., 54
*Haselocke, Jn., B.S., 29
*Hast, Ph., S., 55

92

Printed in the United States
By Bookmasters